Treatment
of
Radiation Injuries

Treatment
of
Radiation Injuries

Edited by

Doris Browne
Joseph F. Weiss
Thomas J. MacVittie
Madhavan V. Pillai

Defense Nuclear Agency
Armed Forces Radiobiology Research Institute
Bethesda, Maryland

Plenum Press • New York and London

Library of Congress Cataloging-in-Publication Data

Consensus Development Conference on the Treatment of Radiation
    Injuries (1st : 1989 : Washington, D.C.)
     Treatment of radiation injuries / edited by Doris Browne ... [et
   al.].
          p.   cm.
     "Proceedings of the First Consensus Development Conference on the
   Treatment of Radiation Injuries, held May 10-13, 1989, in
   Washington, D.C."--T.p. verso.
     Includes bibliographical references.
     Includes index.
     ISBN 0-306-43729-5
     1. Radiation injuries--Treatment--Congresses. 2. Hematopoietic
   system--Radiation injuries--Congresses. 3. Radiation injuries-
   -Complications and sequelae--Congresses.   I. Browne, Doris.
   II. Title.
     [DNLM: 1. Accidents--congresses. 2. Bone Marrow Diseases-
   -therapy--congresses. 3. Growth Substances--therapeutic use-
   -congresses. 4. Infection--congresses. 5. Radiation Injuries-
   -complications--congresses. 6. Radiation Injuries--therapy-
   -congresses. 7. Wounds and Injuries--congresses.   WN 610 C7548t
   1989]
   RC93.C66 1989
   616.9'897--dc20
   DNLM/DLC
   for Library of Congress   90-14216
                                                              CIP

Proceedings of the First Consensus Development Conference on the Treatment of
Radiation Injuries, held May 10-13, 1989, in Washington, D.C.

Views presented in these proceedings are those of the authors; no endorsements by
their organizations have been given or should be inferred.

© 1990 Plenum Press, New York
A Division of Plenum Publishing Corporation
233 Spring Street, New York, N.Y. 10013

Printed in the United States of America

Preface

The proliferation of radioactive materials in industry, in diagnostic and therapeutic medicine, in scientific and medical research, in the military, and as a source of energy has increased the likelihood of accidental exposure to ionizing radiation. Further, the number of individuals exposed in accidents, such as Chernobyl, U.S.S.R.; Goiânia, Brazil; and San Salvador, El Salvador, underscores the potential for large-scale radiation accidents. Because of these accidents, health care providers have found themselves treating patients with acute radiation injuries and subsequent complications. Often the radiation injuries are combined with burns or other trauma and the infectious and immune complications associated with such injuries. The treatment of victims of these accidents has provided important information about the medical management of radiation casualties. However, development of techniques to improve the diagnosis and treatment of radiation injuries, to collect follow-up data on survivors, and to determine the long-term effects of uncontrolled radiation exposure must continue.

The Armed Forces Radiobiology Research Institute, Bethesda, Maryland, and its Medical Radiobiology Advisory Team sponsored the First Consensus Development Conference on the Treatment of Radiation Injuries in Washington, DC, on May 10-13, 1989. The proceedings of the conference are presented in this volume, which we hope will serve as a reference for clinicians and basic research scientists who require knowledge of the latest developments in the diagnosis and treatment of radiation injuries. This conference was designed specifically to address the areas of hematopoietic injury, infectious complications, and combined injury. Other issues pertaining to radiation injuries, such as biologic dosimetry, chemical radioprotection, internal and external radionuclide decontamination, treatment of beta radiation skin burns, potassium iodide prophylaxis, and the development of medical emergency response teams and regional treatment centers, were beyond the scope of this conference and will be addressed at future conferences.

While there have been several significant recent advances in the treatment of infections and burns in immunocompromised patients, this has not been the case with patients sustaining injuries from uncontrolled radiation exposure. Controversy exists regarding the most appropriate techniques in treating the infectious and hematopoietic complications that accompany radiation injuries and/or combined radiation/trauma/burn injuries. A new era in medical radiobiology has dawned. The promise of technological advances in biomedical research generates new insight into the application of this technology to treat individuals with ionizing radiation injuries.

Participants at the consensus conference addressed many factors related to the hematopoietic injury complications of radiation exposure, including bone marrow failure following radiation accidents, the role and use of human recombinant colony-stimulating factors in radiation victims, the use of blood and bone marrow products, bone marrow transplantation, treatment of irradiated animals with recombinant human colony-stimulating factors, and the myeloprotective effects of growth factors.

Additionally, the attendees discussed the infectious complications resulting from radiation injury, including antibiotic, antifungal, and antiviral therapy in neutropenia postirradiation; the role of immunotherapy in preventing infectious complications; treatment of infections in the acute radiation syndrome; prevention of infections with endogenous organisms; and the use of colony-stimulating factors in the Brazilian accident victims. The current status of combined injury and burn management therapy, the implications for healing and infection in the wound environment, and the complications of combined injury in animal models were addressed. These data were correlated to recent radiation accidents.

The consensus statement, developed by the panel of medical and radiobiology experts, evolved from the scientific evidence presented, small group workshops, and roundtable discussions during the conference. Although this consensus statement does not address all aspects of radiation injury, it provides state-of-the-art guidelines for recognizing and treating them.

The editors gratefully acknowledge the contributions of the conference organizing committee; the small group facilitators; the audiovisual support of David H. Morse and Darrell Grant; and the clerical and administrative support staff, especially Darlene Stewart, Judy Kendrick, Gloria Contreras, Mary Jones, Sidney Gibson, Catherine Williams, and Harold Modrow. Our special thanks to the Information Services Department, Armed Forces Radiobiology Research Institute, for its assistance in the development and completion of this book, especially Gloria Ruggiero, Modeste Greenville, Catherine Sund, and Carolyn Wooden. Also, our special thanks to Janet B. Gillette and O. D. Miller for typesetting the text.

Doris Browne

Contents

Appendixes

Hematopoietic Injury Complications

Medical Assessment and Therapy in Bone Marrow Failure Due to Radiation Accidents

Role of Bone Marrow Transplantation and Hematopoietic Growth Factors

Richard Champlin

Introduction

With the increasing use of nuclear energy, it is important that physicians be aware of the principles of managing victims of radiation injuries. This chapter focuses on management of total-body radiation exposure.

The Chernobyl nuclear reactor disaster offers the most graphic description of the risks inherent in nuclear energy. More than 100 million Ci of radioactive materials were released into the environment.[1-3] Victims were exposed to both external and internal sources of radiation. External sources of radiation consisted of beta and gamma radiation emitted from the plume of released radionuclides. Neutron radiation exposure may also occur after nuclear reactor accidents, although it was not an important factor in the Chernobyl accident. Internal radiation exposure includes absorbed, inhaled, or ingested radionuclides. Individuals on the scene of a nuclear accident are usually subjected to skin contamination from airborne radioactive debris.

At Chernobyl, the most seriously affected victims were power plant workers on duty at the time of the accident and firemen called in to control the fires that occurred afterward. They were primarily affected by external radiation, with only minor internal radiation exposure. The population in the surrounding region did not receive doses high enough to cause acute radiation sickness, but individuals were evacuated within a 30-km radius because of concern for long-term health effects.[3]

Cytotoxicity from radiation is dose dependent, and sensitivity varies among cell types and tissues.[4,5] The bone marrow is the critical tissue most sensitive

R. CHAMPLIN, Division of Hematology/Oncology, Department of Medicine, Jonsson Comprehensive Cancer Center, School of Medicine, University of California, Los Angeles, California 90024.

Treatment of Radiation Injuries, Edited by
D. Browne *et al.,* Plenum Press, New York, 1990

to the effects of radiation. With increasing doses, the gastrointestinal (GI) tract, skin, lungs, and other tissues are also affected. In general, cytotoxicity is greatest in rapidly proliferating tissues.[6] Progenitor and precursor cells, such as hematopoietic stem cells of the bone marrow, mucosal crypt cells of the GI tract, and basal epithelial cells of the skin, are more sensitive than mature nonproliferating cells of these tissues.[4,7,8] Because the mature cells of these organs are not lysed by doses typically associated with radiation accidents, the full effects of radiation injury are not manifest until after the preformed cells pass through their normal life span. Maximum organ damage becomes evident as the injured progenitor cells fail to replace the lost mature cells. Lymphocytes are an exception to this rule; they are rapidly lysed by radiation and undergo interphase death. Total-body irradiation rapidly produces profound lymphocytopenia and immunosuppression.[8,9]

The dose-response effects of accidental radiation exposure are poorly defined in humans because of the small number of documented cases in which the size of the absorbed dose could be accurately determined. Radiation injury depends on a number of factors, including the type and quality of radiation, dose, dose rate, homogeneity of the dose, and shielding. Higher doses can be tolerated if given over a protracted time period.[10]

Clinical manifestations of total-body irradiation have been divided into three major dose-related syndromes:[4,5] (1) bone marrow syndrome, (2) GI syndrome, and (3) neurovascular syndrome. Doses of radiation exceeding 1.5-2 Gy produce bone marrow hypoplasia with pancytopenia and immunosuppression, predisposing victims to opportunistic infections and bleeding. The lethal dose (termed $LD_{50/60}$) for 50 percent of individuals within 60 days of total-body irradiation is approximately 4.5 Gy if the victims receive optimal supportive care. Death from bone marrow syndrome generally occurs 14-28 days after exposure from infection in a setting of profound granulocytopenia or thrombocytopenic hemorrhage. The LD_{90} has been estimated to be about 7 Gy.

At higher doses, generally exceeding 8-12 Gy, severe toxicity occurs to the GI tract and other organs. GI syndrome[9] is due to cytotoxicity of the mucosal epithelial cells. High doses of radiation cause loss of the bowel mucosa, massive diarrhea, and sepsis from enteric organisms. Death typically results within 6-9 days. With doses > 8 Gy, pulmonary toxicity also occurs, although symptoms of pneumonitis generally do not develop for 3-7 months.[11] Higher doses of total-body radiation (exceeding 30-50 Gy) produce neurovascular collapse and shock, resulting in death within 2 days.[12]

Cutaneous injury by high-dose beta and gamma radiation produces erythema, epilation, alopecia, and atrophy. These manifestations worsen progressively from 1 to 2 weeks and lead to scaling, wet desquamation, and breakdown, particularly in intertriginous zones.[13] In a nuclear accident, severe associated injuries not directly related to radiation, such as trauma or thermal burns, may occur. Burns substantially increase the mortality of radiation injuries.[14]

The initial therapeutic measure is to prevent further exposure by promptly evacuating victims from the source of radiation. If possible, patients should be rushed to an emergency facility specifically designed to deal with contaminated radiation accident victims.[15-17] Contaminated clothing should be removed and the skin debrided and decontaminated. If radionuclides have been ingested, emetic agents and purgatives should usually be employed. Chelating agents may be useful for some radionuclides.[18] Pulmonary lavage has been proposed after inhalation of plutonium.

After the Chernobyl accident, exposed individuals were not wearing monitoring devices capable of accurately measuring high doses of external radiation. It is, therefore, necessary to estimate the radiation doses based on their biologic effects. Assuming uniform total-body irradiation, several parameters can be used for biologic dosimetry. The earliest indicator is the lymphocyte count; total-body irradiation rapidly produces lymphocytopenia. The rate of fall in circulating lymphocytes is directly related to dose.[19] With doses exceeding 3 Gy, profound lymphocytopenia occurs, and the lymphocyte count is less reliable for estimating the radiation dose.[4,7] Unlike lymphocytes, granulocytes are not directly lysed by radiation. In the bone marrow, there is a large storage pool of granulocytes, which must be mobilized and consumed before granulocytopenia will ensue. The nadir in the granulocyte count typically occurs between 8-30 days after radiation exposure.[8] Higher doses result in increasingly severe granulocytopenia and a shorter interval from exposure to the nadir. The severity of thrombocytopenia and of reticulocytopenia is an indicator of radiation dose, and cytogenetics can also be used to estimate the dose of total-body radiation.[20]

Patients who develop pancytopenia require supportive care similar to that used for bone marrow failure from other etiologies. Infections and bleeding are major causes of morbidity and mortality.[21] Care of skin injuries requires debridement, decontamination, and topical care similar to that necessary for severe thermal burns. Skin grafts may be required.

The GI syndrome is extremely difficult to manage. Diarrhea and fluid depletion must be treated with intravenous fluids and electrolyte replacement. Because oral intake is typically impaired by mucositis and GI intolerance, intravenous hyperalimentation is usually required. Unfortunately, because of damage to the bowel mucosa, severe bleeding and septic shock from enteric organisms generally ensue, and few severely affected patients survive.

Most victims receiving less than 4 Gy total-body irradiation will recover with optimal supportive care. At Chernobyl, 167 of 168 victims who received 1-4 Gy survived. Mortality increases dramatically with higher doses of radiation.

Of the 43 victims who received 4-6 Gy of radiation, 16 survived, and only 1 of 22 victims who received more than 6 Gy survived.[1] Deaths were primarily from bone marrow failure and infection or the GI syndrome.

Role of Bone Marrow Transplantation

It is well documented that bone marrow transplantation can rescue experimental animals and human leukemia patients from lethal total-body irradiation.[22,23] Total-body irradiation produces both immunosuppression and myelosuppression. A sufficiently high dose will prevent rejection of a bone marrow graft. The minimum dose of total-body radiation necessary for engraftment of human bone marrow transplants is poorly defined but exceeds 5 Gy. Engraftment depends on several factors, including the immunologic competence of the recipient; the genetic disparity between donor and recipient; and the source, nature, and number of transplanted hematopoietic cells.[24] In animals, supralethal radiation is required. The risk of graft rejection increases if the donor and recipient are mismatched for major histocompatibility antigens.[25]

Bone marrow transplantation may be associated with many serious complications,[26] particularly graft rejection and graft-versus-host disease. Severe immunodeficiency inevitably occurs for 6-12 months after bone marrow transplantation before immunity is restored by cells derived from the donor bone marrow. Immunosuppressive treatments used to prevent or treat graft-versus-host disease may also produce toxicity and further predispose patients to infection. A variety of serious opportunistic infections may occur. The most frequent fatal infection is cytomegalovirus interstitial pneumonitis. Approximately 30 percent of patients receiving total-body irradiation and bone marrow transplants from HLA-identical donors as treatment for hematologic diseases will die from one or more of these transplant-related complications; the risk of graft rejection and graft-versus-host disease increases substantially with transplants from HLA-nonidentical donors.[27,28]

Bone marrow transplantation is a logical treatment for some victims of accidental total-body irradiation who receive a sufficiently high dose that they are unlikely to have spontaneous marrow recovery. Bone marrow transplantation has many limitations, however, and is likely to benefit only a few patients.[29] Identification of a histocompatible donor is difficult. High-dose total-body irradiation rapidly produces lymphocytopenia, making HLA typing difficult; HLA-A, -B, and -C typing can generally be performed, but insufficient numbers of lymphocytes are usually present to perform mixed lymphocyte culture and HLA-DR typing. The best results have been achieved with transplants from HLA-identical sibling donors, but matched siblings are available for only one-third of victims. Results are also related to age; best results occur in children and young adults. Few patients who are older than 50 years survive bone marrow transplantation. The dose of accidental total-body radiation exposure, although life threatening, may provide insufficient immunosuppression to prevent graft rejection. Using additional immunosuppressive treatments introduces the potential for drug toxicity and increases the risk of opportunistic infections.

At midlethal doses, histoincompatible bone marrow transplantation is associated with increased mortality in mice, a phenomenon termed the "midzone effect" associated with graft rejection.[30] This midzone effect has not been documented in dogs[22,24] or in humans. In other animal models, survival is improved by transplantation of haploidentical T-cell-depleted bone marrow even without sustained engraftment.[31-32] Transient engraftment and hematologic recovery may be protective until autologous marrow recovery occurs.

Victims of nuclear reactor accidents often suffer severe trauma and skin burns in addition to radiation exposure. Most victims of the Chernobyl accident who received a sufficiently high dose of irradiation to be considered for bone marrow transplantation had thermal burns as well as life-threatening radiation injuries to skin, GI tract, lungs, or other tissues. Because of the severe nature of these associated injuries, most of these victims died before enough time had elapsed for a bone marrow transplant to engraft and produce hematologic recovery.[1]

At Chernobyl, 13 victims who had been exposed to more than 5 Gy received bone marrow transplants.[1,33] HLA-identical donors were available for seven patients, and six received related haploidentical transplants. Donors could not be identified for another nine of the most seriously affected patients; these patients received hematopoietic cells from an unrelated fetal liver but died within the next 2 weeks from radiation injuries to the skin, GI tract, and other tissues. Of the 13 bone marrow transplant recipients, 9 had initial engraftment and at least partial recovery of hematopoiesis. Seven died within several weeks from skin burns, GI toxicity, pneumonitis, and infections, and three died from interstitial pneumonitis. Graft-versus-host disease may have contributed to the death of two of these patients. Two transplant recipients survived; each received a haploidentical T-cell-depleted transplant and had transient engraftment of donor cells, followed by recovery of autologous hematopoiesis.

The role of bone marrow transplantation for treatment of nuclear accident victims is controversial. There are no data and few previous experiences to support firm recommendations. Marrow transplantation was performed for four victims of a 1958 nuclear reactor accident in Yugoslavia; these transplants were performed approximately 1 month after exposure, and none of the patients had engraftment.[34] After another accident in 1967, one patient recovered after transplantation of bone marrow from an identical twin; it is impossible to determine if the twin marrow engrafted or if the patient recovered autologous hematopoiesis. The prompt recovery suggested a benefit from transplantation.[35]

Bone marrow transplantation has a limited role for the treatment of victims of radiation accidents. Only a few victims are likely to benefit—those who receive a dose of total-body radiation likely to produce death from bone marrow failure without other life-threatening complications. Given the experience with the Chernobyl victims, transplants should probably be considered only for victims receiving more than 8 Gy of radiation. A number of important factors require further study in animal models, including the optimal interval from exposure to transplantation and the requirement for additional immunosuppressive therapy, particularly for recipients of HLA-nonidentical transplants. The efficacy of T-cell depletion to prevent graft-versus-host disease and the use of unrelated HLA-identical donors for bone marrow transplantation are being evaluated in patients with other hematologic diseases. If techniques can be developed to ensure engraftment without graft-versus-host disease, the efficacy of bone marrow transplantation for radiation victims would be greatly improved.

Hematopoietic Growth Factors

Doses of total-body radiation up to 16 Gy do not completely ablate hematopoiesis. Small numbers of lymphoid cells and hematopoietic progenitors persist,[36,37] although patients receiving > 6 Gy generally succumb to infections or bleeding before hematopoiesis can recover. Recently, several hematopoietic growth factors have been cloned and produced for clinical trials.[38] Granulocyte colony-stimulating factor (G-CSF)[39] and granulocyte-macrophage colony-stimulating factor (GM-CSF)[40] induce leukocytosis in animals and humans.[41,42] Interleukin-3, which stimulates myeloid, erythroid, and megakaryocytic cells, has recently been introduced in clinical trials.[43] These agents stimulate hematopoiesis in patients with aplastic anemia and other bone marrow failure states and increase the rate of hematopoietic recovery after autologous bone marrow transplantation. It is likely that treatment with these agents as single factors or in combinations may enhance the rate of hematopoietic recovery in radiation accident victims and may obviate the need for bone marrow transplantation in high-dose radiation victims. GM-CSF was used to treat severely affected victims in the Goiânia accident, and resulted in improved hematopoiesis.[44] Although the treatment is promising, critical evaluation is necessary to determine if these agents will improve survival of radiation victims with bone marrow failure.

Acknowledgment

This work was supported in part by Grant CA23175 from the National Cancer Institute, National Institutes of Health, Bethesda, Maryland.

References

1. U.S.S.R. State Committee on the Utilization of Atomic Energy. *The Accident at Chernobyl Nuclear Power Plant and Its Consequences.* Presented at the International Atomic Energy Agency Experts Meeting, August 25-29, 1986.
2. U.S. Nuclear Regulatory Commission. *Report on the Accident at the Chernobyl Nuclear Power Station.* NUREG-1250. Washington, DC, 1986.
3. Anspaugh, L. R., Catlin, R. J., and Goldman, M. The global impact of the Chernobyl reactor accident. *Science* 242:1513-1519, 1988.
4. Proceedings of the 35th Session of United Nations Scientific Committee on the Effects of Atomic Radiation. *Early Effects in Man of High Dose Radiation.* Report to the United Nations, 1985.
5. Champlin, R. E., Gale, R. P., and Kastenberg, W. Radiation accidents and nuclear energy: Medical consequences and therapy. *Ann Intern Med* 109:730-734, 1988.
6. Fliedner, T. M., Nothdurft, W., and Steinbach, K. H. Blood cell changes after radiation exposure as an indicator for hemopoietic stem cell function. *Bone Marrow Transplant* 3:77-84, 1988.
7. Bond, V. P., and Cronkite, E. P. Workshop on short-term health effects of reactor accidents: Chernobyl. Report BNL 52030. U.S. Department of Energy, Washington, DC, 1986.
8. Wald, N. Hematological parameters after acute radiation injury. In: *Manual on Radiation Hematology.* International Atomic Energy Agency, Vienna, 1971, pp. 253-264.
9. Wilson, S. G. Radiation-induced gastrointestinal death in the monkey. *Am J Pathol* 35:1233-1251, 1959.
10. Mole, R. H. Quantitative aspects of the lethal action of whole-body irradiation in the human species: Brief and protracted exposure and the applicability of information from other mammalian species. *Int J Radiat Biol* 46:212-213, 1984.
11. Van Dyk, J., Keane, T. J., Kan, S., et al. Radiation pneumonitis following large single dose irradiation: A re-evaluation based on absolute dose to lung. *Int J Radiat Oncol Biol Phys* 7:461-467, 1981.
12. Fanger, H., and Lushbaugh, C. C. Radiation death from cardiovascular shock following a criticality accident: Report of a second death from a newly defined human radiation death syndrome. *Arch Pathol Lab Med* 83:446-460, 1967.
13. Jammet, H., Daburon, F., Gerber, G. B., et al., Eds. Radiation damage to the skin. *Br J Radiol* 19(Suppl), 1986.
14. Brooks, J. W., Evans, E. I., Han, W. T., et al. The influence of external body radiation on mortality from thermal burns. *Ann Surg* 136:533-545, 1952.
15. Shleien, B. *Preparedness and Response in Radiation Accidents.* U.S. Department of Health and Human Services. FDA-HHS No. 83-8211, 1983, pp. 180-195.
16. Saenger, E. L. Radiation accidents. *Ann Emerg Med* 15(9):1061-1066, 1986.
17. Andrews, G. A. Medical management of accidental total-body irradiation. In: *The Medical Basis for Radiation Accident Preparedness.* K. F Hubner and S. A. Fry, Eds. Elsevier North Holland, Inc., New York, 1980, pp. 297-310.
18. Voelz, G. L. Current approaches to the management of internally contaminated persons. In: *The Medical Basis for Radiation Accident Preparedness.* K. F. Hubner and S. A. Fry, Eds. Elsevier North Holland, Inc., New York, 1980, pp. 311-326.
19. Wald, N. Diagnosis and therapy of radiation injuries. *Bull NY Acad Med* 59:1129-1138, 1983.
20. *Biological Dosimetry: Chromosomal Aberration Analysis for Dose Assessment.* Technical Report 260. International Atomic Energy Agency, Vienna, 1986.
21. Bodey, G. P., Buckley, M., Sathe, Y. S., et al. Quantitative relationship between circulating leukocytes and infections in patients with acute leukemia. *Ann Intern Med* 64:328-340, 1966.
22. Monroy, R. L., Vriesendorp, H. M., and MacVittie, T. J. Improved survival of dogs exposed to fission neutron irradiation and transplanted with DLA identical bone marrow. *Bone Marrow Transplant* 2:375-384, 1987.

23. Thomas, E. D., Storb, R., Clift, R. A., *et al.* Bone marrow transplantation. *N Engl J Med* 292:895-902, 1975.

24. Thomas, E. D., LeBond, R., Graham, T., *et al.* Marrow infusions in dogs given sublethal irradiation. *Radiat Res* 41:113-124, 1970.

25. Storb, R., Weiden, P. L., Schroeder, M. L., *et al.* Marrow grafts between canine littermates homozygous or heterozygous for lymphocyte defined histocompatibility antigens. *Transplantation* 21:299-306, 1976.

26. Champlin, R. E., and Gale, R. P. Early complications of bone marrow transplantation. *Semin Hematol* 21:101-108, 1984.

27. Beatty, P. G., Clift, R. A., Michelson, E. M., *et al.* Marrow transplantation from related donors other than HLA-identical siblings. *N Engl J Med* 313:765-771, 1985.

28. Anasetti, C., Amos, D., Beatty, P. G., *et al.* Effect of HLA compatibility on engraftment of bone marrow transplants in patients with leukemia or lymphoma. *N Engl J Med* 320:197-204, 1989.

29. Champlin, R. E. Role of bone marrow transplantation for nuclear accidents: Implications of the Chernobyl disaster. *Semin Hematol* 24(Suppl 2):1-4, 1987.

30. Tretin, J. J. Grafted-marrow-rejection mortality contrasted to homologous disease in irradiated mice receiving homologous bone marrow. *JNCI* 22:219-228, 1959.

31. Ferrera, J., Lipton, J., Hellman, S., *et al.* Engraftment following T-cell depleted marrow transplantation. *Transplantation* 43:461-467, 1987.

32. Lapidot, T., Singer, T. S., and Reisner, Y. Transient engraftment of T-cell depleted allogeneic bone marrow improves survival rate following lethal irradiation. *Bone Marrow Transplant* 3:157-164, 1988.

33. Baranov, A., Gale, R. P., Guskova, A., *et al.* Bone marrow transplantation following the Chernobyl nuclear accident. *N Eng J Med* 321:205-212, 1989.

34. Mathe, G., Jammet, H., Pendic, B., *et al.* Transfusions and homologous bone marrow transplantations in humans accidentally exposed to high doses of radiation. (Transfusions et greffes de moelle ossuese homologue chez des humains irradies a haute dose accidentellement). *Rev Fr Etud Clin Biol* 4:226-238, 1959.

35. Gilberti, M. V. The 1967 radiation accident near Pittsburg, Pennsylvania, and a follow-up report. In: *The Medical Basis for Radiation Accident Preparedness*. K. F. Hubner and S. A. Fry, Eds. Elsevier North Holland, Inc., New York, 1980, pp. 131-140.

36. Butturini, A., Seeger, R., and Gale, R. P. Recipient immune competent T-lymphocytes can survive intensive conditioning for bone marrow transplantation. *Blood* 68:954-956, 1986.

37. Reisner, Y., Ben-Bassat, B., Douer, D., *et al.* Demonstration of clonable alloreactive host T cells in a primate model for bone marrow transplantation. *Proc Natl Acad Sci USA* 83:4012-4015, 1986.

38. Clark, S. C., and Kamen, R. The human hematopoietic colony-stimulating factors. *Science* 236:1229-1237, 1987.

39. Souza, L. M., Boone, T. C., Gabrilove, J., *et al.* Recombinant human granulocyte-colony stimulating factor: Effects on normal and leukemic myeloid cells. *Science* 232:61-65, 1986.

40. Metcalf, D. The granulocyte-macrophage colony-stimulating factors. *Science* 229:16-22, 1985.

41. Gabrilove, J. L., Jakubowski, A., Scher, H., *et al.* Effect of granulocyte colony-stimulating factor on neutropenia and associated morbidity due to chemotherapy for transitional cell carcinoma of the urothelium. *N Engl J Med* 318:1414-1422, 1988.

42. Champlin, R., Nimer, S. D., Ireland, P., *et al.* Treatment of refractory aplastic anemia with recombinant human granulocyte-macrophage colony-stimulating factor. *Blood* 73:694-699, 1989.

43. Yang, Y. C., Ciarletta, A. B., Temple, P. A., *et al.* Human IL-3 (multi-CSF): Identification by expression cloning of a novel hematopoietic growth factor related to murine IL-3. *Cell* 47:3-10, 1986.

44. Butturini, A., DeSouza, P. C., Gale, R. P., *et al.* Use of recombinant granulocyte-macrophage colony stimulating factor in the Brazil radiation accident. *Lancet* II:471-475, 1988.

Use of rhGM-CSF in Bone Marrow Failure

Is There a Therapeutic Role for GM-CSF
in Accidental Radiation Injuries?

Joseph H. Antin

Introduction

Radiation accidents resulting in significant injury are, fortunately, uncommon. However, one of the primary manifestations of radiation injury is bone marrow suppression. Depending on the dose of radiation and the manner in which it is received, hematologic effects can be acute and severe or chronic and delayed. The manifestations include aplastic anemia as well as increased risk of leukemia.

Hematopoietic growth factors have been suggested as potentially useful agents to ameliorate hematopoietic injury from radiation.[1,2] The recent cloning, expression, and production of large amounts of several hematopoietic growth factors have resulted in an opportunity to study the effects of growth factors in patients with normal and abnormal hematopoiesis. These observations may allow some insights into potential benefits and problems to be expected from growth-factor therapy of radiation-induced marrow injury.

Erythropoietin was the first growth factor successfully applied to human marrow dysfunction.[3] It was clearly demonstrated that the anemia arising from failure of renal production of erythropoietin could be reversed by the exogenous administration of the protein. It was reasoned that a similar benefit might be derived from growth factors that had been shown *in vitro* to be necessary for hematopoiesis. Early studies of the granulocyte-macrophage colony-stimulating factor (GM-CSF) in nonhuman primates[4] rapidly gave rise to trials in myelodysplastic syndrome (MDS),[5-7] aplastic anemia,[6,8-10] and idiopathic agranulocytosis,[6,11] and after intensive chemotherapy administered for autologous marrow transplantation[12,13] or treatment of malignancies.[14] Unfortunately, our understanding of the complex interactions of stimulatory

J. H. ANTIN, Division of Hematology, Department of Medicine, Brigham and Women's Hospital, Boston, Massachusetts 02115.

Treatment of Radiation Injuries, Edited by
D. Browne *et al.,* Plenum Press, New York, 1990

and inhibitory cytokines in the day-to-day control of hematopoiesis is slim, and growth factors have been applied to the treatment of patients before their physiologic role was carefully elucidated.

Rationale

Patients with persistent marrow failure due to aplastic anemia and MDS have received attention as potential beneficiaries of growth-factor therapy. Transient bone marrow failure from chemotherapy will not be considered in this discussion, because spontaneous improvement is expected. Aplastic anemia is the result of a heterogeneous group of pathophysiologic events that result in an overall reduction in hematopoiesis. A proportion of these patients have immunologically mediated marrow failure, but many have a reduction in the total number of hematopoietic stem cells and progenitors. In addition, a small proportion of patients with marrow aplasia have microenvironmental abnormalities that prevent hematopoiesis. It is possible that some of these individuals have aplastic anemia by virtue of deficient growth-factor production by abnormal or abnormally regulated lymphoid cells or by disordered cytokine production by the marrow stroma.

Patients with MDS have disordered hematopoiesis, which is usually clonal. The genes coding for many of the growth factors (for example, GM-CSF and interleukin-3 (IL-3)) are located on the long arm of chromosome 5, an area that is often involved in chromosomal aberrations in myelodysplasia. The relationship between chromosome 5 abnormalities, clinical MDS, and hematopoietic growth factors is intriguing but unclear.

Mortality is high among patients with aplastic anemia who cannot undergo marrow grafting and who are unresponsive to antithymocyte globulin therapy. With the exception of marrow transplantation, there are no effective treatments for patients with MDS. The profound pancytopenia that is characteristic of these disorders eventually results in death from infection, bleeding, iron overload, or leukemic conversion. Studies of these patients were undertaken to assess both the toxicity of parenterally administered GM-CSF and the likelihood of clinical benefit from marrow stimulation.

Methods

Recombinant human GM-CSF was administered to patients with MDS, aplastic anemia, and idiopathic agranulocytosis in four protocols: (1) daily 1-hour intravenous infusions for 7 days; (2) daily 4-hour infusions for 7 days; (3) daily 12-hour infusions for 14 days; and (4) daily 24-hour infusions for 14 days.[5-10] Patients were eligible for further therapy with or without dose modifications. The doses were not strictly comparable because two different preparations were used, and they had different specific activities. Furthermore, some doses were based on body weight and others on body surface area. The GM-CSF provided by Immunex Corporation (Seattle, WA) was produced in yeast[15] and contained a leucine substituted for an arginine at position 23 to facilitate production by yeast. The other formulation was provided by Sandoz (East Hanover, NJ) and was produced in mammalian COS cells.[16]

Aplastic Anemia and Agranulocytosis

Five studies reported the results of treatment of 34 patients with aplastic anemia or agranulocytosis with GM-CSF.[6,8-11] Most of the patients had severe transfusion-dependent aplastic anemia. Bone marrow biopsy demonstrated ≤ 15 percent cellularity in 33 patients and < 25 percent cellularity in 1 patient with aplastic anemia from paroxysmal nocturnal hemoglobinuria.

The responses to treatment were heterogeneous. Although transient increases in granulocytes from twofold to greater than tenfold were often observed, several patients had little or no increase in any hematopoietic cell population. None of the reported patients had any improvement in platelets, and none had sustained improvement in hematopoiesis. Responses of granulocytes, monocytes, and reticulocytes were observed in many patients, regardless of their dosing regimen. However, when GM-CSF was administered by continuous infusion, even higher absolute neutrophil counts were sometimes achieved, often in association with striking eosinophilia.

It was difficult to demonstrate a dose-response relationship because the subjects' initial hematologic status and treatment regimens were heterogeneous. Although increases in granulocyte and monocyte counts were observed at the lowest doses used, reticulocyte responses were more frequently observed at the higher dose levels. The UCLA group noted more extreme leukocytosis with increasing doses, but often the leukocytosis was due in large part to eosinophils.[10]

Two of the three patients with idiopathic agranulocytosis had no responses to GM-CSF infusion in any cell line. The third patient had a dramatic response of granulocytes to the 12-hour infusion of GM-CSF at 240 μg/m^2/day (J. H. Antin, unpublished data). The patient developed severe bone discomfort, which required a 50-percent reduction in dosage. Unfortunately, the response abated immediately with the discontinuation of GM-CSF.

Myelodysplastic Syndrome

Three studies evaluated GM-CSF in the treatment of MDS. These studies are also difficult to compare because of the heterogeneity of patients with

MDS, the different regimens used, and the inclusion of patients with primary as well as secondary disease.[5-7] Treatment regimens were similar to those described for aplastic anemia.

Of the 34 patients with MDS who were reported, 29 had primary MDS and 5 had marrow dysfunction due to chemotherapy. In general, a more dramatic increase of blood cells was observed in the patients with MDS than in the aplastic patients. Twofold to fifteenfold increases in neutrophils, monocytes, and eosinophils were routinely observed, as well as increases in reticulocytes in some patients. A reduction in transfusion requirement for red blood cells or platelets apparently occurred in three individuals.

Toxicity

Toxicity of GM-CSF can be divided into effects that appear to be dose related and effects that are independent of dose (table 1). The predominant complaints not related to dose were low back or rib discomfort, anorexia, myalgias and arthralgias, and low-grade fever. The low back discomfort was severe enough to require analgesia in some patients. Anaphylactic reactions were observed (J. H. Antin, unpublished observations). Patients who noted a side effect with one administration of GM-CSF tended to have it again with subsequent administrations. There did not appear to be a significant difference in dose-independent toxicity between the 1-hour, 4-hour, 12-hour, and 24-hour infusions.

Dose-related side effects included fluid retention, thrombophlebitis, pericarditis, and pulmonary infiltrates.[10,12,14] These effects were often severe and dose limiting. It was unclear whether the difference in toxicity was related to the product. Patients in the Sandoz-sponsored studies appeared to be more likely to develop pericarditis and thrombosis, but they tended to get higher

Table 1. Toxicity of GM-CSF Infusions

Independent of dose	Related to dose
Bone discomfort	Eosinophilia
Myalgias and arthralgias	Pulmonary infiltrates
Fever	Fluid retention
Headache	Pericarditis
Anorexia	Thrombosis
Nausea and vomiting	Stimulation of leukemic
Muscle twitching	blasts
Fatigue	
Anaphylaxis	
Marrow fibrosis	
Inhibition of neutrophil migration	

doses of GM-CSF.[9,10,12,14] Recent studies have demonstrated GM-CSF receptors on endothelial cells, suggesting that some of the toxicities may be mediated through a direct vascular effect. We did not detect any antibodies to GM-CSF in any of the six patients tested, although all patients tested had multiple exposures to the protein.

A problem unique to the myelodysplastic patients was leukemic cell stimulation, resulting in temporary increases in myeloblasts in some individuals but leukemic conversion in others.[7] This effect was seen only in patients with chronic myelomonocytic leukemia, refractory anemia with excess blasts (RAEB), or RAEB in transition.

A group of 10 patients with MDS was treated at the Brigham and Women's Hospital with 240 μg/m^2/day for 14 days. Three of these patients developed increases in bone marrow fibrosis in association with the GM-CSF therapy.[17] Concomitant reductions in neutrophils and platelets were observed in one individual as well. The hematologic status of these patients did not seem to worsen dramatically. The etiology of this unexpected problem is uncertain, but it may be related to stimulation of megakaryocytes, endothelial cells, or other marrow stromal elements, with the subsequent production of additional cytokines, such as platelet-derived growth factor, fibroblast growth factor, or β-transforming growth factor, which might stimulate collagen deposition.

One additional problem deserves mention. Peters *et al.* convincingly demonstrated a reduction in migration of granulocytes into skin in patients who received continuous infusions of GM-CSF.[18] This effect is less prominent if the GM-CSF is administered intermittently. Although no infectious complications have been ascribed to neutrophil migration inhibition, such complications are a concern in patients who are already immunocompromised. This effect might be particularly problematic if accidental radiation exposure was associated with trauma, burns, or radiation skin injuries.

Role of Hematopoietic Growth Factors in Accidental Radiation Injury

High-dose ionizing radiation can produce marrow aplasia in a dose-dependent fashion. This result is largely due to direct injury of stem cells and progenitors by the radiation, but effects on the marrow microenvironment are also possible. Low-dose or intermittent therapeutic radiation is a common cause of MDS in patients treated for nonhematopoietic malignancies. Clinical studies of patients with marrow failure have led to the following conclusions: GM-CSF administered by continuous infusion or intermittent infusion can substantially increase the neutrophil count and monocyte count in most, but not all, patients with marrow failure. Patients with the most severe depression of hematopoiesis appear the least likely to respond. GM-CSF does not consistently increase the reticulocyte or platelet counts. Few patients had any reduction in transfusion requirements, and these improvements might have reflected spontaneous remissions. Toxicity appears to be acceptable, but concerns about the stimulation of leukemic cell growth, marrow fibrosis, and inhibition of granulocyte egress into the tissues raise questions about the risks of clinical use of GM-CSF. Any benefits from GM-CSF in increasing the granulocyte count are short lived. The drug must be used for brief periods of time to overcome a self-limited period of myelosuppression, or it must be given indefinitely. The risks of long-term use are uncertain.

What is the role of GM-CSF in the therapy of radiation accidents? GM-CSF was administered to eight patients in Brazil after accidental exposure to ~2.5 Gy to 6 Gy of internal and external radiation from cesium-137.[2] Four of the patients survived the injury, and the others died of bacterial sepsis or hemorrhage. Although GM-CSF infusion increased the neutrophils in five patients, its role in the survival of four of these individuals is unclear. As expected from observations in nonirradiated patients, there was no effect on erythrocytes or platelets.

The risk of poor neutrophil migration into areas of thermal injury or trauma necessitates caution in the use of GM-CSF in this setting. Granulocyte colony-stimulating factor (G-CSF) will increase the neutrophil count, and does not affect neutrophil migration. If neutropenia is the primary clinical concern, G-CSF might be a more appropriate agent. IL-1, IL-3, and IL-6 are other hematopoietic growth factors that may stimulate earlier cells in the hematopoietic differentiation pathway; however, studies of their effects in humans are just beginning. In nonhuman primates, combinations of GM-CSF and IL-3 are synergistic, allowing neutrophilia at doses that should not inhibit granulocyte migration.[19] Perhaps combined growth-factor therapy will allow more accurate stimulation of stem cell compartments and avoid some of the problems associated with stimulation of the function of mature cells.

There may be additional risks to the use of growth factors in this setting. Our lack of knowledge about the interactions of GM-CSF and other growth factors with irradiated marrow warrants caution in the clinical use of these agents. Do growth factors provide a proliferative stimulus that will act synergistically with the mutagenic stimulus of irradiation and accelerate the development of leukemia? Most clinical settings are inadequate models to address this question. Therapeutic irradiation for marrow grafting is given by external irradiation rather than by a combination of external and internal irradiation, and the new marrow is not irradiated. If there has been significant radioisotope ingestion, there may be continued irradiation of the marrow while the proliferative stimulus is present. The predominant isotopes causing the injury are extremely important. One might anticipate particular problems with isotopes such as strontium-90, which may irradiate the marrow for long periods. Although there is no evidence of stem cell depletion as a consequence of

GM-CSF therapy, other growth factors (for example, IL-1 and IL-6) may have effects on resting stem cells; if these cells are brought into the cell cycle during irradiation, cytotoxic and mutagenic effects might be more severe.

There is a dearth of clinical information on which to base recommendations regarding the treatment of radiation-accident-induced marrow injury. The answers to these questions will require the development of animal models as well as increased understanding of the effects of growth factors in humans.

Acknowledgment

This study was supported in part by a grant from the M. Larry Lawrence Foundation and by grants from the National Institutes of Health.

References

1. Champlin, R. E. Radiation accidents and nuclear energy: Medical consequences and therapy. *Ann Intern Med* 109:730-744, 1988.
2. Butturini, A., DeSouza, P. C., Gale, R. P., *et al.* Use of recombinant granulocyte-macrophage colony-stimulating factor in the Brazil radiation accident. *Lancet* 2:471-475, 1988.
3. Esbach, J. W., Egrie, J. C., Downing, M. R., *et al.* Correction of the anemia of end-stage renal disease with recombinant human erythropoietin. Results of a combined phase I and II clinical trial. *N Engl J Med* 316:73-78, 1987.
4. Donahue, R. E., Wang, E. A., Stone, D. K., *et al.* Stimulation of haematopoiesis in primates by continuous infusion of recombinant human GM-CSF. *Nature* 321:872-875, 1986.
5. Vadhan-Raj, S., Keating, M., LeMaistre, A., *et al.* Effects of recombinant human granulocyte-macrophage colony-stimulating factor in patients with myelodysplastic syndromes. *N Engl J Med* 317:1545-1552, 1987.
6. Antin, J. H., Smith, B. R., Holmes, W., *et al.* Phase I/II study of recombinant human granulocyte-macrophage colony-stimulating factor in aplastic anemia and myelodysplastic syndrome. *Blood* 72:705-713, 1988.
7. Ganser, A., Volkers, B., Greher, J., *et al.* Recombinant human granulocyte-macrophage colony-stimulating factor in patients with myelodysplastic syndromes: A phase I/II trial. *Blood* 73:31-37, 1989.
8. Vadhan-Raj, S., Buescher, S., Broxmeyer, H. E., *et al.* Stimulation of myelopoiesis in patients with aplastic anemia by recombinant human granulocyte-macrophage colony-stimulating factor. *N Engl J Med* 319:1628-1634, 1988.
9. Nissen, C., Tichelli, A., Gratwohl, A., *et al.* Failure of recombinant human granulocyte-macrophage colony-stimulating factor therapy in aplastic anemia patients with very severe neutropenia. *Blood* 72:2045-2047, 1988.
10. Champlin, R. E., Nimer, S. D., Ireland, P., *et al.* Treatment of refractory aplastic anemia with recombinant human granulocyte-macrophage colony-stimulating factor. *Blood* 73:694-699, 1989.
11. Thomassen, C., Nissen, C., Gratwohl, A., *et al.* Agranulocytosis associated with T-gamma-lymphocytosis: No improvement of peripheral blood granulocyte count with human-recombinant granulocyte-macrophage colony-stimulating factor. *Br J Haematol* 71:157-160, 1989.
12. Brandt, S. J., Peters, W. P., Atwater, S. K., *et al.* Effect of human granulocyte-macrophage colony-stimulating factor on hematopoietic reconstitution after high-dose chemotherapy and autologous bone marrow transplantation. *N Engl J Med* 318:869-876, 1988.

13. Neumunaitis, J., Singer, J. W., Buckner, C. D., *et al.* Use of recombinant human granulocyte-macrophage colony-stimulating factor in autologous marrow transplantation for lymphoid malignancies. *Blood* 72:834-836, 1988.
14. Antman, K. S., Griffin, J. D., Elias, A., *et al.* Effect of recombinant human granulocyte-macrophage colony-stimulating factor on chemotherapy-induced myelosuppression. *N Engl J Med* 319:593-598, 1988.
15. Cantrell, M. A., Anderson, D., Ceretti, D. P., *et al.* Cloning, sequence, and expression of a human granulocyte-macrophage colony-stimulating factor. *Proc Natl Acad Sci USA* 82:6250-6254, 1985.
16. Wong, G. G., Witek, J. S., Temple, P. A., *et al.* Human GM-CSF: Molecular cloning of the complementary DNA and purification of the natural and recombinant proteins. *Science* 228:810-815, 1985.
17. Antin, J. H., Weinberg, D. S., and Rosenthal, D. S. Variable effect of recombinant human granulocyte-macrophage colony-stimulating factor on bone marrow fibrosis in patients with myelodysplasia. *Exp Hematol*, in press.
18. Peters, W. P., Stuart, A., Affronti, M. L., *et al.* Neutrophil migration is defective during recombinant human granulocyte-macrophage colony-stimulating factor infusion after autologous bone marrow transplantation in humans. *Blood* 72:1310-1315, 1988.
19. Donahue, R. E., Seehra, J., Metzger, M., *et al.* Human IL-3 and GM-CSF act synergistically in stimulating hematopoiesis in primates. *Science* 241:1820-1823, 1988.

Blood and Bone Marrow Products in the Treatment of Radiation Injury

C. Robert Valeri

Introduction

The recent nuclear accidents at Chernobyl, U.S.S.R., and Goiânia, Brazil, have heightened concerns about the immediate availability of personnel, facilities, equipment, blood, and blood products for treating individuals exposed to radiation. The proper diagnosis and treatment of individuals exposed to radiation depend on methods used to detect the type and magnitude of radiation exposure, to decontaminate both the individuals and the environment (for example, animals, food, and water), and to monitor individual radiation exposure to identify individuals who will require blood and bone marrow products.

Radiation injures bone marrow hematopoietic stem cells, producing leukopenia, thrombocytopenia, and anemia. The bleeding disorder associated with thrombocytopenia requires treatment with viable and functional platelets, and the resulting anemia may require red blood cell transfusion. Depending on the magnitude of the radiation injury, bone marrow transplantation with pluripotential stem cells also may be required. Because radiation immunosuppresses the patient, it is necessary to irradiate the donor platelet concentrates, red blood cells, and plasma to inactivate the viable immunocompetent lymphocytes and prevent graft-versus-host disease.[1,2] Hematopoietic growth factors that stimulate the residual endogenous stem cells should be administered to stimulate production of red cells, platelets, and granulocytes-macrophages.[3-17] Colony-stimulating factors (CSF's) that activate granulocytes and macrophages, granulocytes, megakaryocytes, and red blood cells (recombinant human erythropoietin) are being investigated for possible new drug applications.[3-17]

Pluripotential stem cells can be isolated from bone marrow and peripheral blood. During the collection of bone marrow, the individual is subjected to

C. R. VALERI, Naval Blood Research Laboratory, 615 Albany Street, Boston, Massachusetts 02118.

Treatment of Radiation Injuries, Edited by
D. Browne *et al.,* Plenum Press, New York, 1990

general anesthesia, and about 500 to 600 mL of blood containing bone marrow cells are collected. Morbidity is associated with the collection of bone marrow from 50 to 100 aspiration sites. There is only minimal morbidity associated with the isolation of pluripotential stem cells from peripheral blood, and the procedure is relatively simple. Peripheral blood contains about 10-15 percent as many pluripotential mononuclear cells as bone marrow. Eight to ten apheresis procedures are needed to obtain an adequate number of mononuclear cells from peripheral blood.

Under ideal conditions, red blood cells should be ABO and Rh compatible and irradiated to inactivate any viable immunocompetent lymphocytes.[1] Platelets should be ABO and HLA compatible, devoid of white blood cells (which may produce alloimmunization), and irradiated to inactivate any viable immunocompetent lymphocytes. The allogeneic pluripotential stem cells should be ABO and HLA compatible and devoid of immunocompetent lymphocytes to prevent graft-versus-host disease in the irradiated immuno-suppressed recipient.

Medical personnel and proper facilities are needed to test healthy blood donors; to isolate multiple units of platelets and pluripotential mononuclear cells from donors, using mechanical apheresis equipment; and to obtain ABO- and HLA-compatible bone marrow from anesthetized individuals. Healthy donors of blood products and bone marrow must be tested for ABO, Rh, and HLA antigens; syphilis; hepatitis B antigen; antibodies to human immunodeficiency virus, human T-cell lymphotrophic virus-type I (HTLV-I), and hepatitis B core antigen; and the serum alanine aminotransferase level.

Frozen Blood Banks Containing Red Blood Cells, Platelets, Fresh Frozen Plasma, and Pluripotential Stem Cells

The blood products required to properly treat individuals exposed to radiation should be stockpiled: universal donor O-positive and O-negative irradiated red blood cells, pools of compatible irradiated frozen platelets, irradiated fresh frozen AB plasma, and ABO- and HLA-compatible pluripotential stem cells that are devoid of immunocompetent cells and have been isolated from peripheral blood mononuclear cells of healthy volunteers.

Platelets and red blood cells are resistant to radiation injury, whereas pluripotential stem cells are sensitive to radiation injury.[1] Pluripotential stem cells must be properly shielded during frozen storage to protect them from radiation injury. The Department of Defense has mandated the deployment of frozen blood banks by the U.S. Army, Navy, and Air Force. The frozen blood bank system uses -80°C mechanical refrigerators to freeze (1) universal donor O-positive and O-negative red blood cells in original 800-mL polyvinylchloride plastic bags, (2) pools of 6 to 8 units of ABO-compatible platelets that have been obtained from units of whole blood or by plateletpheresis of healthy volunteers, using mechanical apheresis instruments, and frozen in polyvinylchloride plastic bags, and (3) universal donor AB plasma.[18,19]

Human red blood cells are frozen with 40 percent weight/volume glycerol and can be stored at -80°C for at least 21 years with excellent results.[20] To date, the Food and Drug Administration (FDA) has authorized the storage of red cells containing 40 percent weight/volume glycerol at -80°C for only 10 years. Previously frozen red blood cells contain a small number of residual viable immunocompetent lymphocytes after thawing and washing,[21] and it is not known whether these cells might produce graft-versus-host disease in an immunosuppressed recipient. It has been recommended by some investigators that all deglycerolized red blood cells be irradiated.

Deglycerolized red blood cells can be stored in a sodium-chloride-glucose solution at 4°C for at least 3 days with freeze-thaw-wash recovery of about 90 percent, 24-hour posttransfusion survival of at least 80 percent, only slightly reduced oxygen transport function, and minimal residual hemolysis.[20] However, FDA has approved storage of the deglycerolized red cells at 4°C for only 24 hours because the systems used in the deglycerolization process are not closed, and sterile docking devices are not currently used.

Pools of 6 to 8 units of ABO-compatible platelets obtained from units of whole blood or from healthy volunteers by plateletpheresis procedures are frozen within 6-8 hours of collection and stored at 22°C ± C 2°C.[19,22] Preliminary data indicate that it is safe to store pools of 6 to 8 units of platelets at 22°C ± 2°C for 24 hours before freezing. FDA approval of this extended storage period would provide adequate time to perform the mandated testing of the platelets for infectious agents before freezing.

A pool of 6 to 8 units of platelets is frozen with 6 percent dimethylsulfoxide (DMSO) in plasma at 2°C to 4°C per minute in a polyvinylchloride plastic bag in an aluminum container placed in a -80°C mechanical freezer.[19,22] Preliminary data from studies evaluating a disposable plastic tray to replace the aluminum container indicate that a freezing rate of 2°C to 4°C per minute can be achieved by storing the plastic container in a -80°C mechanical freezer with a fan to circulate the air in the chamber. The platelets can be frozen and stored at -80°C for up to 2 years.[19] After thawing, the platelets can be washed to remove 95 percent of the DMSO, resuspended in acid-citrate-dextrose (ACD) plasma, and stored at 22°C for 6 hours. About 75-80 percent of the platelets are recovered after the freeze-thaw-wash procedure. About 30-35 percent of the infused platelets are recovered *in vivo*, and these platelets have a normal lifespan and are hemostatically effective within 2-4 hours after infusion.

Approximately 2.5 units of liquid preserved or cryopreserved platelets are needed to achieve the same number of circulating platelets in the recipient as 1 unit of fresh platelets.[19,22] In aspirinated baboons, a prolonged bleeding time was corrected immediately after the transfusion of fresh platelets. Cryopreserved platelets corrected the bleeding time in aspirinated baboons during the 2- to 4-hour posttransfusion period, but the 5-day-old platelets did not.

Our data show that frozen, universal donor AB plasma can be stored at -80°C for at least 2 years. FDA has approved the storage of fresh frozen plasma at -20°C for only 1 year.

Irradiation of Platelet Concentrates, Red Blood Cell Concentrates, and Plasma to Inactivate the Viable Immunocompetent Lymphocytes

Red blood cells and platelets are resistant to radiation injury.[23,24] Viable and functional lymphocytes are contained in fresh blood; liquid-preserved whole blood and red blood cell concentrates; previously frozen, washed red blood cells; fresh frozen plasma; fresh platelet concentrates; liquid-preserved platelet concentrates; and previously frozen, washed platelets.[1] These blood products should be irradiated to inactivate the viable immunocompetent lymphocytes. Gamma irradiation of the blood products with a dose of 20-50 Gy has been recommended to abolish the mitotic activity of the lymphocytes without adversely affecting the red blood cells, platelets, and plasma proteins.[25-30]

Freeze Preservation of Peripheral Blood and Bone Marrow Pluripotential Stem Cells

During the past 6 years, the Naval Blood Research Laboratory (NBRL) has been evaluating the cryopreservation of peripheral blood and bone marrow pluripotential mononuclear cells obtained from healthy volunteers.[31] By the use of mechanical cell separators, the mononuclear cells are obtained from the cellular residue remaining after the plateletpheresis procedure. By means of a Ficoll-Hypaque procedure in a plastic bag system, designed and developed at NBRL, mononuclear cells are isolated from the cellular residue.[32] The same procedure has been used to isolate autologous mononuclear cells from bone marrow obtained from anesthetized patients with solid tumors. Autologous bone marrow stem cells are frozen for subsequent use.[33]

Mononuclear cells obtained from peripheral blood or bone marrow are isolated by Ficoll-Hypaque gradient centrifugation, washed to remove the Ficoll-Hypaque gradient, and then frozen with 10-percent DMSO in plasma at 2°C to 4°C per minute in polyvinylchloride plastic bags or polyolefin plastic bags stored in aluminum containers or provials; they are then frozen in a mechanical freezer maintained at -80°C to control the rate of freezing.[34,35] The mononuclear cells frozen in the polyvinylchloride plastic bags were stored at -80°C in a mechanical freezer, and the mononuclear cells frozen in polyolefin plastic bags were stored at -135°C in a mechanical freezer. A volume of 40 mL containing 15 million mononuclear cells per mL was frozen in polyvinylchloride and polyolefin plastic bags. The provials were stored in the mechanical freezers maintained at -80°C and -135°C, in the gas phase of liquid nitrogen at -150°C, or in the liquid phase of liquid nitrogen at -197°C. A volume of 2 mL containing 15 million cells per mL was frozen in the provials.

The frozen mononuclear cells were thawed and washed with a sodium-chloride-glucose-phosphate solution, pH 5.0, and resuspended in ACD plasma. Measurements were made of freeze-thaw-wash recovery, membrane integrity of the mononuclear cells assessed using ethidium bromide and fluorescein diacetate, and growth of the mononuclear cells in the granulocyte-erythrocyte-macrophage/monocyte-megakaryocyte colony-forming unit (GEMM-CFU) assay.[36] In one assay, the mononuclear cells were stimulated with phyto-hemagglutinin-lymphocyte-conditioned medium. In another assay, the mononuclear cells were stimulated with irradiated human leukocytes. The results of the two methods were similar, and the results were combined and averaged. Mononuclear cells ranging from 32 x 10^3, 64 x 10^3, and 128 x 10^3 were plated, and the number of GEMM-CFU per 10^5 mononuclear cells was reported. The GEMM-CFU assay was performed on the fresh mononuclear cells before and after the addition of DMSO, after thawing, and after washing.[35] The overall freeze-thaw-wash recovery was 90 percent, and the membrane integrity assessed by ethidium bromide and fluorescein diacetate was about 90 percent. In the mononuclear cells frozen in the polyvinylchloride plastic bags stored at -80°C and in the polyolefin plastic bags stored at -135°C for 1 year, thawed, and washed, the growth was similar to the fresh mononuclear cells.

Studies are in progress to assess mononuclear cells frozen with 10-percent DMSO in provials and stored for more than 1 year at -80°C, -135°C, -150°C, and -197°C; in polyvinylchloride plastic bags at -80°C; and in polyolefin plastic bags stored at -135°C. Polyvinylchloride plastic bags tolerate storage at -80°C but break when stored at -135°C; polyolefin plastic bags, on the other hand, tolerate storage at both -80°C and -135°C. Studies will be done to determine whether deterioration occurs in mononuclear cells preserved with 10-percent DMSO and stored for more than 1 year at -80°C in polyvinylchloride plastic bags or at -135°C in polyolefin plastic bags.

It is important that the immunocompetent lymphocytes present in mono-nuclear cells obtained from peripheral blood and bone marrow be removed to avoid graft-versus-host disease. Treatment with monoclonal antibodies and lectin agglutination and rosetting with sheep erythrocytes have been used with some success.[33] Simpler methods are needed, however, and studies are in progress toward this end.

In our laboratory, we removed the granulocytes and red cells by Ficoll-Hypaque treatment and froze only the isolated mononuclear cells. In previous studies, in which nucleated cells containing white blood cells and red blood cells were not removed before freezing of the mononuclear cells at -80°C, deterioration was reported.[37,38] If we find deterioration after prolonged storage at -80°C, we will store the mononuclear cells at -135°C in polyolefin plastic bags in a mechanical freezer. We prefer to store the frozen mononuclear cells in the -80°C mechanical freezer used to freeze preserve red blood cells, platelets, and fresh frozen plasma; our second choice is the -135°C mechanical freezer. We recommend storing frozen cells and plasma in mechanical freezers because they do not require liquid nitrogen, which is expensive and difficult to transport.

Frozen autologous platelets and peripheral blood mononuclear cells that have been obtained by plateletpheresis procedures using mechanical cell separation instruments can now be stockpiled in nuclear submarines and nuclear power plants. It is much easier to isolate peripheral blood mononuclear cells than it is to collect bone marrow by aspiration. In specific clinical situations, mechanical apheresis procedures provide large numbers of autologous or allogeneic pluripotential stem cells that can be used in combination with bone marrow stem cells.

Summary

Radiation injures the bone marrow hematopoietic stem cells, resulting in leukopenia, thrombocytopenia, and anemia. The bleeding disorder associated with thrombocytopenia requires treatment with platelets and sometimes with red blood cells. Depending on the magnitude of the radiation injury, bone marrow or peripheral blood hematopoietic stem cells may be required.

This chapter discusses the availability and use of random-donor and HLA-compatible-donor fresh, liquid-preserved, and cryopreserved platelets, HLA-compatible fresh and cryopreserved bone marrow stem cells, and fresh and cryopreserved hematopoietic stem cells devoid of immunocompetent stem cells obtained from peripheral blood. Irradiation of platelet concentrates, red cell concentrates, and fresh frozen plasma is recommended to inactivate the viable immunocompetent lymphocytes present in these blood products to prevent graft-versus-host disease in the immunocompromised recipient exposed to radiation. Viable and functional platelets are needed to treat the bleeding disorder produced by the thrombocytopenia. HLA-compatible bone marrow stem cells may be required to treat the bone marrow aplasia, and

CSF's may be needed to stimulate the endogenous stem cells to produce granulocytes-macrophages, platelets, and red blood cells.

Peripheral blood mononuclear cells obtained as a by-product during plateletpheresis procedures can be isolated by Ficoll-Hypaque gradient centrifugation; these cells contain pluripotential stem cells that grow in the GEMM-CFU tissue culture assay. The immmunocompetent lymphocytes must be removed to prevent graft-versus-host disease in the recipient. Pluripotential stem cells obtained from bone marrow and peripheral blood can be frozen with 10-percent DMSO at 2°C to 4°C per minute and stored at -80°C in polyvinylchloride plastic bags or at -135°C in polyolefin plastic bags for at least 1 year.

Allogeneic peripheral blood mononuclear cells devoid of immunocompetent lymphocytes, as well as red blood cells, platelets, and fresh frozen plasma, can be frozen to build a stockpile for use in the event of a nuclear accident.

Acknowledgment

Research was supported by the U.S. Navy (Office of Naval Research Contract N00014-79-C-0168, with funds provided by the Naval Medical Research and Development Command). The opinions and assertions contained in this chapter are those of the author and are not to be construed as official or reflecting the views of the Navy Department or Naval Service at large.

The author acknowledges the secretarial assistance of Ms. Gina Ragno and the editorial assistance of Ms. Cynthia Valeri.

References

1. Valeri, C. R. *Blood Banking and the Use of Frozen Blood Products.* Chemical Rubber Company, Boca Raton, Florida, 1976.
2. Park, B. H., Good, R. A., Gate, J., *et al.* Fatal graft-vs-host reaction following transfusion of allogeneic blood and plasma in infants with combined immunodeficiency disease. *Transplant Proc* 6:385-387, 1974.
3. Donahue, R. E., Wang, E. A., Stone, D. K., *et al.* Stimulation of haematopoiesis in primates by continuous infusion of recombinant human GM-CSF. *Nature* 321:872-875, 1986.
4. Eschbach, J. W., Egrie, J. C., Downing, M. R., *et al.* Correction of the anemia of end-stage renal disease with recombinant human erythropoietin. Results of a combined phase I and II clinical trial. *N Engl J Med* 316:73-78, 1987.
5. Mayer, P., Lam, C., Obenaus, H., *et al.* Recombinant human GM-CSF induces leukocytosis and activates peripheral blood polymorphonuclear neutrophils (PMNs) in non-human primates. *Blood* 70:206-213, 1987.
6. Gillio, A. P., Bonilla, M. A., Potter, G. K., *et al.* Effects of recombinant human granulocyte colony-stimulating factor on hematopoietic reconstitution after autologous bone marrow transplantation in primates. *Transplant Proc* 19:153-156, 1987.
7. Groopman, J. E., Mitsuyasu, R. T., DeLeo, M. J., *et al.* Effect of recombinant human granulocyte-macrophage colony-stimulating factor on myelopoiesis in the acquired immunodeficiency syndrome. *N Engl J Med* 317:593-598, 1987.

8. Matsumoto, M., Matsubara, S., Matsuno, T., *et al.* Protective effect of human granulocyte colony-stimulating factor on microbial infection in neutropenic mice. *Infect Immun* 55:2715-2720, 1987.

9. McDonald, T. P., Cottrell, M. B., Clift, R. E., *et al.* High doses of recombinant erythropoietin stimulate platelet production in mice. *Exp Hematol* 15:719-721, 1987.

10. Monroy, R. L., Skelly, R. R., MacVittie, T. J., *et al.* The effect of recombinant GM-CSF on the recovery of monkeys transplanted with autologous bone marrow. *Blood* 70:1696-1699, 1987.

11. Nienhuis, A. W., Donahue, R. E., Karlsson, S., *et al.* Recombinant human granulocyte-macrophage colony-stimulating factor (GM-CSF) shortens the period of neutropenia after autologous bone marrow transplantation in a primate model. *J Clin Invest* 80:573-577, 1987.

12. Antman, K. S., Griffin, J. D., Elias, A., *et al.* Effect of recombinant human granulocyte-macrophage colony-stimulating factor on chemotherapy-induced myelosuppression. *N Engl J Med* 319:593-598, 1988.

13. Berridge, M. V., Fraser, J. K., Carter, J. M., *et al.* Effects of recombinant human erythropoietin on megakaryocytes and on platelet production in the rat. *Blood* 72:970-977, 1988.

14. Brandt, S. J., Peters, W. P., Atwater, S. K., *et al.* Effect of recombinant human granulocyte-macrophage colony-stimulating factor on hematopoietic reconstitution after high-dose chemotherapy and autologous bone marrow transplantation. *N Engl J Med* 318:869-876, 1988.

15. Griffin, J. D. Clinical applications of colony-stimulating factors. *Oncology* 2:15-21, 1988.

16. Monroy, R. L., Skelly, R. R., Taylor, P., *et al.* Recovery from severe hematopoietic suppression using recombinant human granulocyte-macrophage colony stimulating factor. *Exp Hematol* 16:344-348, 1988.

17. Peters, W. P., Stuart, A., Affronti, M. L., *et al.* Neutrophil migration is defective during recombinant human granulocyte-macrophage colony-stimulating factor infusion after autologous bone marrow transplantation in humans. *Blood* 72:1310-1315, 1988.

18. Valeri, C. R., Sims, K. L., Bates, J. F., *et al.* An integrated liquid-frozen blood banking system. *Vox Sang* 45:25-39, 1983.

19. Valeri, C. R. Cryobiology. In: *Methods in Hematology: Blood Transfusion, Vol. 17.* T. J. Greenwalt, Ed. Churchill Livingstone, Edinburgh, U.K., 1988, pp. 277-304.

20. Valeri, C. R., Pivacek, L. E., Gray, A. D., *et al.* The safety and therapeutic effectiveness of human red cells stored at -80°C for as long as 21 years. *Transfusion* 29:429-437, 1989.

21. Crowley, J. P., Skrabut, E. M., and Valeri, C. R. Immunocompetent lymphocytes in previously frozen washed red cells. *Vox Sang* 26:513-517, 1974.

22. Valeri, C. R. The current state of platelet and granulocyte cryopreservation. *CRC Crit Rev Clin Lab Sci* 14:21-74, 1981.

23. Schiffer, L. M., Atkins, H. L., Chanana, A. D., *et al.* Extracorporeal irradiation of the blood in humans: Effect upon erythrocyte survival. *Blood* 27:831-843, 1966.

24. Greenberg, M. L., Chanana, A. D., Cronkite, E. P., *et al.* Extracorporeal irradiation of blood in man: Radiation resistance of circulating platelets. *Radiat Res* 35:147-154, 1968.

25. Button, L. N., DeWolf, W. C., Newburger, P. E., *et al.* The effects of irradiation on blood components. *Transfusion* 21:419-426, 1981.

26. Leitman, S. F., and Holland, P. V. Irradiation of blood products. Indications and guidelines. *Transfusion* 25:293-300, 1985.

27. Moore, G. L., and Ledford, M. E. Effects of 4000 rad irradiation on the *in vitro* storage properties of packed red cells. *Transfusion* 25:583-585, 1985.

28. Holland, P. V., and Schmidt, P. L., Eds. *Standards for Blood Banks and Transfusion Services.* 12th ed., American Association of Blood Banks, Arlington, Virginia, 1987.

29. Read, E. J., Kodis, C., Carter, C. S., *et al.* Viability of platelets following storage in the irradiated state: A pair-controlled study. *Transfusion* 28:446-450, 1988.

30. Rock, G., Adams, G. A., and Labow, R. S. The effects of irradiation on platelet function. *Transfusion* 28:451-455, 1988.

31. Valeri, C. R. Cryopreservation of human platelets and bone marrow and peripheral blood totipotential mononuclear stem cells. *Ann NY Acad Sci* 459:353-366, 1986.

32. Carciero, R., and Valeri, C. R. Isolation of mononuclear leukocytes in a plastic bag system using Ficoll-Hypaque. *Vox Sang* 49:373-380, 1985.
33. Krupp, K. R., Lowder, J. N., and Herzig, R. H. Bone marrow processing for transplantation. In: *Methods in Hematology: Blood Transfusion, Vol. 17.* T. J. Greenwalt, Ed. Churchill Livingstone, Edinburgh, U.K., 1988, pp. 257-276.
34. Valeri, C. R., Melaragno, A. J., Dittmer, J., et al. *Bone Marrow Reconstitution of Lethally Irradiated Beagles by Treatment With Autologous Previously Frozen Bone Marrow or Peripheral Blood Mononuclear Cells Obtained as a Byproduct of Plateletpheresis.* Naval Blood Research Laboratory/Boston University School of Medicine, Technical Report No. 85-01, Boston, MA, 1985.
35. Valeri, C. R., Ragno, G., Gray, A., et al. *Cryopreservation of Mononuclear Cells Isolated From the Peripheral Blood of Human Volunteers: Effects of the Cryoprotectant Solution (10% DMSO-Plasma or 5% DMSO-6% HES-4% HSA), the Rate of Freezing (1°C/minute or 2-4°C/minute), and the Temperature of Storage in the Frozen State (-80°C or -150°C) for 3 Months on the In Vitro Recovery of Mononuclear Cells and Their Growth in the GEMM-CFU Tissue Culture Assay.* Naval Blood Research Laboratory/Boston University School of Medicine, Technical Report No. 86-02, Boston, MA, 1986.
36. Horland, A., Ziegelstein, R., Carciero, R., et al. *Comparison of Human and Baboon Marrow Mononuclear Cells in GEMM-CFU Tissue Culture System.* Naval Blood Research Laboratory/ Boston University School of Medicine, Technical Report No. 85-04, Boston, MA, 1985.
37. Malinin, T. I., Pegg, D. E., Perry, V. P., et al. Long-term storage of bone marrow cells at liquid nitrogen and dry ice temperatures. *Cryobiology* 7:65-69, 1970.
38. O'Grady, L. F., and Lewis, J. P. The long-term preservation of bone marrow. *Transfusion* 12:312-316, 1972.

Total-Body Irradiation in Bone Marrow Transplantation

Rainer Storb, H. Joachim Deeg,
Frederick R. Appelbaum,
Friedrich G. Schuening, Robert Raff,
and Theodore Graham

Introduction

The exquisite sensitivity of lymphohematopoietic tissues to ionizing radiation has been known since shortly after the discovery of x rays by Roentgen. The most prominent features of the hematopoietic syndrome in experimental animals are hemorrhagic complications and susceptibility to infections. Since the late 1940's it has been known that the hematopoietic radiation injury could be modified by subsequent infusion of bone marrow. By the mid-1950's, three independent groups of investigators showed that the lifesaving effect of marrow infusions was due to the presence of pluripotent stem cells in the transplant, from which regrowth of the damaged hematopoietic system occurred.

The implications of these observations reach far beyond the problem of modifying radiation injury. The fact that grafted marrow cells persist in irradiated recipients offers a variety of therapeutic possibilities, not only for the patients involved in a radiation accident, but also for the patients with leukemia and acquired or inherited dysfunction of the hematopoietic system.

The goal of total-body irradiation (TBI) in the treatment of patients with hematological malignancies is to deliver the greatest possible immunosuppressive effect (to allow acceptance of the foreign marrow graft) and the greatest possible anticancer effect, with the least possible toxicity to nonhematopoietic tissues. At least three variables may alter the effects of TBI: total radiation dose, radiation dose rate, and dose fractionation. It may be possible to alter these variables to gain greater immunosuppressive and anticancer effects with

---

R. STORB and F. R. APPELBAUM, Clinical Research Division, Fred Hutchinson Cancer Research Center, 1124 Columbia Street, Seattle, Washington 98104, and University of Washington School of Medicine, 1959 NE Pacific Street, Seattle, Washington 98105; F. G. SCHUENING, R. RAFF, and T. GRAHAM, Clinical Research Division, Fred Hutchinson Cancer Research Center, 1124 Columbia Street, Seattle, Washington 98104; H. J. DEEG, University of British Columbia and Vancouver General Hospital, 910 W. 10th Avenue, Vancouver, British Columbia V52 4E3.

Treatment of Radiation Injuries, Edited by
D. Browne *et al.,* Plenum Press, New York, 1990

less toxicity. Radiobiological studies carried out in isolated tissues and in mice suggest that the effect on the marrow would be the same for a given total dose of single or fractionated TBI, whereas sparing of nonhematopoietic tissues would be accomplished by dose fractionation (provided that fractions were spaced 3-6 hours apart).

This chapter provides a review of our TBI studies with a random-bred preclinical canine model and addresses marrow toxicity, nonhematopoietic organ toxicity, and immunosuppressive effects of single-dose versus fractionated radiation in the context of marrow transplantation. TBI was delivered from two opposing cobalt-60 sources. During the postirradiation period, canines were given parenteral fluid and electrolyte support, broad-spectrum antibiotics, oral nonabsorbable antibiotics, and red blood cell and platelet transfusions subjected to 1,500 cGy *in vitro* irradiation to inactivate lymphocytes.

Marrow Toxicity of TBI

We explored the marrow toxicity of single-dose TBI delivered at a rate of 10 cGy/minute and compared results to those seen with TBI administered in 100-cGy fractions with minimum fractionation intervals of 6 hours.[1] We found that 200-cGy single-dose TBI was sublethal; the eight canines so treated showed hematopoietic recovery and survived. Only 4 of 11 canines given 300-cGy single-dose TBI survived, and none of 5 canines given 400 cGy survived. By comparison, 6 of 11 canines given 300-cGy TBI in three fractions survived, and none of 5 canines given 400 cGy in four fractions survived.

Thus, survival among canines given single-dose versus fractionated-dose TBI was not different (p = 0.8). Also, the slopes of the postirradiation declines of granulocyte and platelet counts in canines given single-dose versus fractionated TBI were indistinguishable. We concluded that, within the limitations of the experimental design, single-dose and fractionated TBI have comparable marrow toxicity in canines.

Nonhematopoietic Organ Toxicity

In these studies, 113 canines were given TBI, followed by grafts of cryopreserved autologous marrow to prevent death from marrow toxicity.[2,3] Acute and delayed nonhematopoietic toxicities of single-dose and fractionated TBI given at various total doses and delivered at 2.1, 5, 10, and 20 cGy/min were compared. A logistic regression analysis of the data indicated that the type of delivery (single-dose versus fractionated TBI) has only suggestive significance with regard to the acute toxicity (p = 0.054), whereas both total dose (p = 0.005) and dose rate (p < 0.001) are important. For example, a dose rate of 5 cGy/min permitted administration of an additional 400 cGy of TBI than delivery at 10 cGy/min (1,400 cGy versus 1,000 cGy) did, and more canines receiving 1,400 cGy at 10 cGy/min died than canines given 1,000 cGy at the same dose rate. Theoretical expectations of a benefit of fractionation on gastrointestinal toxicity were not fulfilled, perhaps with the exception of canines given TBI at 20 cGy/min. Further studies at higher dose rates per minute are needed to clarify this issue.

Nonhematopoietic toxicity of canines given fractionated versus single-dose TBI was comparable, but differences emerged with regard to late toxicities. For example, among canines that survived the period of early acute gastrointestinal toxicity, survival was best after fractionated TBI. Approximately 85 percent of canines given fractionated TBI became long-term survivors, compared to only 5 percent of canines given single-dose TBI. Causes of death included wasting syndrome, hepatic failure, pancreatic fibrosis, and development of hypoproliferative anemia.

Immunosuppressive Effects of TBI

We explored the ability of single-dose versus fractionated TBI, given at a rate of 7 cGy/min at otherwise lethal doses of 450, 600, 700, 800, and 920 cGy, to condition canines for marrow grafts from dog-leukocyte-antigen-identical (DLA-identical) littermates.[4,5] We found that fractionated TBI was less immunosuppressive than single-dose TBI; the evidence was a significantly higher rate of graft rejection (p = 0.001). Specifically, sustained marrow engraftment was seen in only 2 of 18 canines (11 percent) given 600-800 cGy of fractionated TBI, compared to 11 of 17 canines (65 percent) given comparable doses of single-dose TBI. Only at 450 cGy (none of the 10 canines studied had sustained engraftment) and at 920 cGy (4 of 5 canines given fractionated TBI and 20 of 21 canines given single-dose TBI engrafted) were we unable to find differences between the two modes of radiation. Most canines that rejected their grafts survived with subsequent autologous hematopoietic recovery (13 of 22 given fractionated TBI and 8 of 12 given single-dose TBI; p = 0.49). Recovery was presumably the result of extended support provided by the transient allogeneic grafts. We concluded that, at equivalent doses, fractionated TBI was significantly less effective than single-dose TBI in conditioning DLA-identical littermate canines for marrow grafting.

These findings have implications for the design of conditioning programs used in clinical transplantation, especially when T-cell-depleted marrow grafts are employed. If these data are extrapolated to the human patient who has experienced a radiation accident, we conclude that marrow grafts from siblings identical for the major histocompatibility complex are beneficial in the setting of otherwise lethal radiation exposures. We anticipate that most individuals would either experience sustained allogeneic grafts or survive with autologous marrow recovery because of the blood cell support provided by a transient allogeneic graft.

Although DLA-identical marrow grafts are generally successful following 920 cGy of TBI, allografts are largely unsuccessful following this dose of TBI when marrow is infused from DLA-nonidentical (unrelated or littermate) donors.[6,7] Presumably, resistance to a DLA-nonidentical graft is caused by lymphoid cells surviving the high dose of TBI. Successful grafts in the DLA-nonidentical setting were seen only after 1,800 cGy of TBI had been delivered in three 600-cGy fractions over a period of 4 days.

Use of rhG-CSF After TBI

In view of reported attempts to overcome marrow failure after a radiation accident by treating victims with a recombinant hematopoietic growth factor, we explored the effect of recombinant human granulocyte colony-stimulating factor (rhG-CSF) on endogenous marrow recovery in canines after otherwise lethal TBI.[8] RhG-CSF given subcutaneously at 10 or 100 μg/kg/day for 2 weeks raises peripheral blood neutrophils eightfold to tenfold and monocytes fourfold to sixfold above controls in normal canines. Lymphocyte counts increased threefold at the higher dose of rhG-CSF. No significant changes were observed in eosinophil, platelet, reticulocyte, or hematocrit levels. After 2 weeks of treatment with rhG-CSF, marrow showed hyperplasia and left-shifting of the granulocytic line. After discontinuation of rhG-CSF, peripheral leukocyte counts returned to control levels within 3 days.

In the current study, five canines given 400-cGy TBI at 10 cGy/minute and no marrow infusion or growth factor all developed profound pancytopenia and died between 17 and 23 days after TBI with infections secondary to marrow aplasia. Four of five canines treated within 2 hours of 400-cGy TBI with 100 μg rhG-CSF/kg/day subcutaneously twice a day for 21 days showed complete and sustained endogenous hematopoietic recovery and survived. In contrast, five canines irradiated with 400-cGy TBI and treated with 100 μg rhG-CSF/kg/day starting on day 7 after TBI all died with infections between days 17 and 20 after TBI. Thus, it appears that rhG-CSF, if begun shortly after TBI, can reverse the otherwise lethal myelosuppressive effect of radiation exposure.

We do not know yet whether the beneficial effect of rhG-CSF can be improved by combining it with other growth factors, such as interleukin-3, which is thought to stimulate earlier hematopoietic progenitor cells. Also, we do not know whether treatment with hematopoietic growth factors will be consistently effective after higher TBI exposures.

Acknowledgment

This work was supported by grants CA18221, CA18029, CA31787, CA18105, and CA15704 of the National Cancer Institute, National Institutes of Health, U.S. Department of Health and Human Services.

References

1. Thomas, E. D., LeBlond, R., Graham, T., *et al.* Marrow infusions in dogs given midlethal or lethal irradiation. *Radiat Res* 41:113-124, 1970.
2. Deeg, H. J., Storb, R., Weiden, P. L., *et al.* High dose total body irradiation and autologous marrow reconstitution in dogs: Dose rate related acute toxicity and fractionation dependent long-term survival. *Radiat Res* 88:385-391, 1981.
3. Deeg, H. J., Storb, R., Longton, G., *et al.* Single dose or fractionated total body irradiation and autologous marrow transplantation in dogs: Effects of exposure rate, fraction size, and fractionation interval on acute and delayed toxicity. *Int J Radiat Oncol Biol Phys* 15:647-653, 1988.
4. Storb, R., Raff, R. F., Appelbaum, F. R., *et al.* What radiation dose for DLA-identical canine marrow grafts? *Blood* 72:1300-1304,1988.
5. Storb, R., Raff, R. F., Appelbaum, F. R., *et al.* Comparison of fractionated to single dose total body irradiation in conditioning canine littermates for DLA-identical marrow grafts. *Blood* 74:1139-1143, 1989.
6. Deeg, H. J., Storb, R., Shulman, H. M., *et al.* Engraftment of DLA-nonidentical unrelated canine marrow after high-dose fractionated total body irradiation. *Transplantation* 33:443-446, 1982.
7. Storb, R., and Deeg, H. J. Failure of allogeneic canine marrow grafts after total body irradiation: Allogeneic "resistance" versus transfusion induced sensitization. *Transplantation* 42:571-580, 1986.
8. Schuening, F. G., Storb, R., Goehle, S., *et al.* Effect of recombinant human granulocyte colony-stimulating factor on hematopoiesis of normal dogs and on hematopoietic recovery after otherwise lethal total body irradiation. *Blood* 74:1308-1313,1989.

Rescue of Lethally Irradiated Animals

Therapeutic Use of rhG-CSF and rhGM-CSF in Preclinical Models of Radiation-Induced Marrow Aplasia

Thomas J. MacVittie and Rodney L. Monroy

Introduction

Three recent radiation accidents—the reactor explosion in Chernobyl, U.S.S.R.,[1] the external and internal cesium-137 exposure in Goiânia, Brazil,[2] and the cobalt-60 exposure of three technicians in El Salvador, San Salvador—exemplify the usual conditions of accidental radiation exposure. The exposure environment is ill defined and uncontrolled.[3] The radiation delivery is heterogeneous and nonuniform, and may vary in rate, quality, and energy. It is the uncontrolled nature of the radiation exposure, in addition to the potential for shielding, that forecasts the possible sparing of cells essential for survival, i.e., the stem cells of the hematopoietic system and the gastrointestinal system. Radiation experiments in which areas of the bone marrow were shielded have demonstrated the potential of spared bone marrow cells to repopulate the hematopoietic tissue and to increase not only the production of granulocytes and platelets but also the chances of surviving an otherwise lethal dose of radiation.[4-11]

The advent of recombinantly produced and purified hematopoietic growth factors and cytokines has shown significant promise for the development of therapeutic protocols. Experimental evidence using purified cytokines in mice,[12-24] canines,[25-31] and nonhuman primates[25,32-38] has provided new and interesting possibilities in therapeutic enhancement of stem cell and progenitor cell recovery. Most of these studies, however, have dealt with inducing recovery in animals after sublethal exposure to drugs or radiation. Survival following lethal doses of radiation requires (1) renewal of hematopoietic stem cells that have been reduced to levels that normally will not support survival, and (2)

T. J. MacVITTIE, Department of Experimental Hematology, Armed Forces Radiobiology Research Institute, Bethesda, Maryland 20814-5145; R. L. MONROY, Immunobiology and Transplantation Branch, Naval Medical Research Institute, Bethesda, Maryland 20814-5055.

Treatment of Radiation Injuries, Edited by
D. Browne *et al.*, Plenum Press, New York, 1990

production of functional end cells (granulocyte and platelet) within a critical, clinically manageable time period necessary to prevent hemorrhage and infection from opportunistic pathogens.

Recently, Schuening and his colleagues[30] have shown that therapeutic administration of recombinant human granulocyte colony-stimulating factor (rhG-CSF) will rescue canines from an otherwise 100-percent lethal dose of radiation. We have also recently shown that administering recombinant human granulocyte-macrophage colony-stimulating factor (rhGM-CSF) or rhG-CSF to primates and canines after lethal doses of radiation will not exhaust a severely depleted stem cell population and will induce earlier recovery of granulocytes and platelets and increase survival.

Materials and Methods

Domestic-born male rhesus monkeys (*Macaca mulatta*, mean weight 3.1 kg ± 0.2 kg) and purpose-bred canines (beagles, mean weight 10.0 kg ± 0.4 kg) were housed in individual stainless-steel cages in conventional holding rooms of the AAALAC-accredited animal facility at the Armed Forces Radiobiology Research Institute (AFRRI). Monkeys and canines were provided 10 air changes per hour of 100-percent fresh air, conditioned to 72°F ± 2°F with relative humidity of 50 percent ± 20 percent, and were maintained on a 12-hour light/ dark full-spectrum light cycle with no twilight. Monkeys and canines were provided tap water *ad libitum* and commercial primate and canine chow, with the addition of fresh fruit for the monkeys. Research was conducted according to the principles enunciated in the *Guide for the Care and Use of Laboratory Animals*, prepared by the Institute of Laboratory Animal Resources, National Research Council.

Monkeys were exposed to a nonuniform, nonhomogeneous dose of cobalt-60 radiation as previously described.[37] In brief, chair-adapted, unanesthesized monkeys were exposed to opposing cobalt-60 sources while restrained in a Plexiglas chair. Lead walls shielded the tibia without causing a change in dose to the torso and head (figure 1; table 1). Midline tissue dose at navel height was delivered to a total of 800 cGy at a dose rate of 500-735 cGy/minute. Measured midline tissue doses for head, torso, femur, and tibia are shown in table 1. The shielding effectively reduced the dose to the tibia and femur by 47 percent and 27 percent, respectively, from the torso dose of 800 cGy.

Canines were bilaterally exposed to uniform, homogeneous, total-body cobalt-60 radiation at a dose rate of 40 cGy/minute to total doses of 200, 300, 350, 400, and 450 cGy at midline tissue. Radiation exposure took place in well-ventilated Plexiglas restraint boxes (after prior acclimatization).

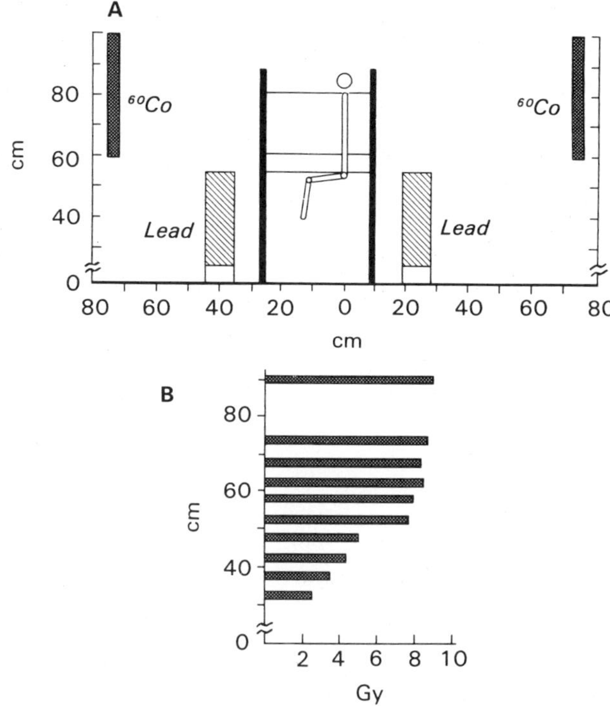

Figure 1. (A) Exposure array with monkey, chair, shield, and source. The lead walls (44 cm wide by 31 cm high by 8.8 cm thick) were placed on a wood base. The asymmetry of the center of the monkey to the lead walls was a limitation imposed by the structure of the restraint chair. (B) Free-in-air dose distribution versus height.

The rhGM-CSF (Genetics Institute, Cambridge, MA) used in the primate studies had an activity of 10^7 U/mL (6.25×10^6 U/mg). A unit of activity for rhGM-CSF was defined as the amount of rhGM-CSF needed to stimulate a half-maximal incorporation of ^{3}H-thymidine by chronic-myelogenous-leukemia peripheral blood myeloblasts.

The rhG-CSF (Amgen, Thousand Oaks, CA) used in these studies was produced with *Escherichia coli* according to recombinant DNA techniques. This agent was at least 95-percent pure, was formulated in an aqueous buffer, and had no measurable endotoxin determined by the limulus amebocyte assay. The specific activity of the recombinant protein was 1×10^8 or more units per milligram of protein.[39]

Table 1. Distribution and Dose of Radiation Received
Following Nonuniform Exposure to 800 cGy

Body region	Marrow distribution (percent of total)[1]	Mean midtissue dose (cGy)[2]
Tibia	5.9	425
Femur	13.3	584
Torso	69.9	800
Head	10.9	896

[1]Rhesus monkey bone marrow distribution. Source: Taketa, S. T., Carsten, A. L., Cohn, S. H., *et al.* Active bone marrow distribution in the monkey. *Life Sci* 9:169-174, 1970.
[2]Phantoms were seated between two lead walls, providing partial shielding to the tibia during exposure.

The rhGM-CSF and rhG-CSF were administered to the monkeys as previously described.[37] In brief, the monkeys received rhGM-CSF subcutaneously via implanted osmotic minipumps at a rate of 72,000 U/kg/day over a period of 7 days, following a single dose of 50,000 U/kg administered intravenously on day 3 or day 4 after radiation exposure. The canines received rhGM-CSF (Genetics Institute, Cambridge, MA, or Amgen, Thousand Oaks, CA) subcutaneously in two equally divided doses for a total 100 μg/kg/day and rhG-CSF in one dose of 10 μg/kg/day. Therapeutic administration of each factor began on day 1 after exposure and continued for 14 consecutive days in the sublethally exposed (200 cGy) canines and 21-24 consecutive days in the lethally exposed canines.

Bone-marrow-derived granulocyte-macrophage colony-forming cells (GM-CFC) and peripheral blood GM-CFC's were assayed in monkey and canine tissue as described previously.[40,41] In brief, the double-agar assay technique was used with rhGM-CSF as the stimulating factor for each species, with the addition of giant cell-tumor-conditioned medium for the monkey marrow cultures and the addition of endotoxin-stimulated sera for the canine marrow cultures.

Clinical and experimental manipulations of the monkeys have been described.[37,40] Animals were clinically monitored daily. The canine support regimen consisted of antibiotics initiated when the white blood cell count fell below 100/mm³, and was maintained until the count rose above that level and remained there for 3 consecutive days. A combination of gentamycin sulfate (3 mg/kg, twice daily intramuscularly) and cefotaxime sodium (claforan: load dose of 30 mg/kg intramuscularly; twice daily dose of 30 mg intramuscularly) was used. Fresh, irradiated platelets (1,500 cGy, random donor) were administered when the platelet count dropped below 40,000/mm³. At signs of dehydration, 20 mL/kg of Ringer's lactate was administered in a slow intravenous drip into the lateral cephalic vein (for 1 hour), with 20 mL/kg/day administered subcutaneously.

Results

The radiation models were designed to induce certain degrees of lethality in the clinically supported animals. The radiation dose associated with a certain lethality could then be correlated with a percentage of surviving, marrow-derived progenitor cells—in this case, the GM-CFC—assuming that the stem cell has a radiation sensitivity not significantly different from the GM-CFC (approximately 75 cGy, D_0). In this way the percentage of surviving stem cells can be associated with the inability to support survival. Lethality implies that the stem cell cannot renew itself to a level that can support differentiation into lifesaving granulocytes and platelets before hemorrhage and/or infection cause death, that is, within a clinically manageable time period. It is at these levels of stem cell survival that we evaluated the therapeutic efficacy of rhGM-CSF and rhG-CSF.

A uniform, total-body dose of 800 cGy to an unshielded, fully supported monkey is 100-percent lethal; the total fraction of surviving bone-marrow-derived stem cells is estimated to be less than 0.00001. The approximate $LD_{50/30}$ for the clinically supported rhesus monkey is 525 cGy,[42] or a surviving stem cell fraction of approximately 0.0007. We calculated the surviving fraction of stem cells in our shielded monkeys to be approximately 0.001, a value that should translate into lethality for the exposed monkeys. The experimentally determined lethality was 20 percent, a value lower than expected, but which may have been the combined result of expert clinical support, effective antibiotics, and housing in an AAALAC-accredited facility. Treatment with rhGM-CSF from day 3 to day 11 did not change survival (four of five monkeys survived with or without rhGM-CSF therapy), but showed a significant effect on decreasing the period of neutropenia and thrombocytopenia. The one rhGM-CSF-treated monkey that did not survive also showed signs of hematopoietic recovery, whereas the untreated monkey that did not survive remained aplastic.

The shielded control monkeys reached granulocyte levels greater than 1,000/ mm³ on day 22, whereas the 7 days of rhGM-CSF treatment induced recovery of granulocytes above this level by day 18, or 4 days earlier (figure 2A). Platelet production also responded to rhGM-CSF treatment. Platelet levels were depressed through day 24 in the untreated monkeys, whereas treatment with rhGM-CSF induced recovery as early as day 18 to day 20 (figure 2B).

The effect of rhGM-CSF treatment on recovery of marrow-derived GM-CFC was evident at earlier times in both the iliac crest and the tibia. The results were more pronounced in the iliac crest, where the concentration of GM-CFC

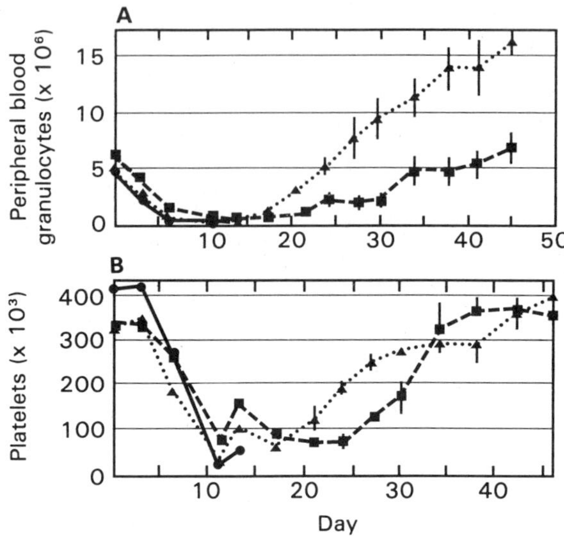

Figure 2. Effect of shielding with rhGM-CSF treatment on the recovery of (A) peripheral blood granulocytes and (B) platelets in monkeys. Each point is a mean ± SEM for the groups: unshielded (—•—), shielded (--■--), and shielded with treatment (· · · ▲ · · ·).

in rhGM-CSF-treated monkeys increased more than tenfold in comparison to that of the control (saline-treated) shielded monkeys (table 2).

This preliminary model of severe radiation-induced marrow aplasia and stem cell depletion illustrated that 7 days of therapeutic rhGM-CSF administration

Table 2. Effect of rhGM-CSF Treatment on the Recovery of GM-CFC[1] Derived From Iliac Crest Marrow

Days[2]	Control	rhGM-CSF
3	0	0
10	0	8±4
20	2±1	18±2
31	55±18	65±20
40	58±15	80±24

[1]GM-CFC per 10^5 mononuclear cells, mean value ± SEM.
[2]Time in days after 800-cGy midline cobalt-60 irradiation of shielded monkeys.

will significantly reduce the period of neutropenia and thrombocytopenia through earlier regeneration of marrow-derived progenitor cells. It was also apparent that initiation of treatment on day 3 after radiation exposure would not exhaust a severely depleted stem cell population and thereby induce greater lethality.

Both rhGM-CSF and rhG-CSF elicited a rapid and sustained granulopoietic response throughout the period of administration. The rhG-CSF was significantly more active than the rhGM-CSF on a weight basis; one-tenth the amount of rhG-CSF (10 μg/kg) produced almost twice the level of leukocytosis that rhGM-CSF produced at 100 μg/kg (figure 3). These levels of leukocytosis were associated with hypercellular marrow and an increased granulopoietic differential. Both rhG-CSF and rhGM-CSF induced a significant rise in the concentration of marrow-derived GM-CFC and were also active *in vitro* in supporting proliferation of GM-CFC in clonogenic, agar-supported assays.

RhG-CSF and rhGM-CSF were tested in both sublethal and lethal radiation models in therapeutic protocols consisting of consecutive, daily administration initiated 1 day after exposure and continued for 14 days or 21-24 days, depending on the exposure dose. Both factors were effective in diminishing the severity and period of neutropenia in sublethally irradiated canines and in significantly shortening the severity and period of neutropenia in canines lethally irradiated at an $LD_{60/30}$ dose (350 cGy).

Administration of rhG-CSF or rhGM-CSF to the high-dose sublethally irradiated canines produced a prompt release of marrow-resident reserve

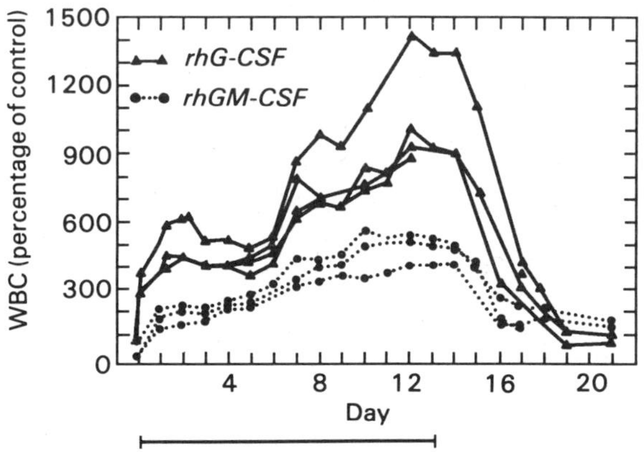

Figure 3. Increase in peripheral white blood cells (WBC) after injections of 10 μg/kg/day of rhG-CSF and 100 μg/kg/day of rhGM-CSF for 14 consecutive days. Each data point represents one experimental canine.

granulocytes over the first several days (figure 4). Peripheral leukocytes dropped to levels near those of irradiated controls, followed by a sustained production of granulocytes throughout the duration of the injection protocol (day 15). The production of granulocytes to greater than normal levels was associated with increased marrow cellularity and concentration of GM-CFC. Cessation of the treatment protocol resulted in a decrease of white cells to a level within normal baseline range throughout the observation period. This decrease indicated a completely recovered population of granulopoietic progenitor cells capable of maintaining normal granulocyte production while the marrow in irradiated controls was still in its recovery phase. The dramatic success at inducing recovery in the 200-cGy-irradiated canines with these recombinant human CSF's prompted continued evaluation at higher lethal radiation doses.

Irradiation of a canine to a total midline tissue dose of 350 cGy is always lethal without complete clinical support consisting of fluids, antibiotics, and fresh irradiated platelets; with clinical support, it is a lethal dose for 60 percent of the exposed animals ($LD_{60/30}$). The percentage survival of marrow-derived GM-CFC is reduced to approximately 1 percent of normal. The increase in survival (40 percent) is a consequence of increased hematopoietic regeneration during the extended survival time afforded by the clinical support. Mean survival time increased from 14 days to 20 days. The extra 6 days allow the surviving stem cells and progenitor cells critical time for self-renewal and production of granulocytes. The recombinant CSF's in this case act as multiplying factors, using the extra time (when the animal is free of infection from opportunistic pathogens) to generate an increased fraction of progenitor cells large enough to produce enough granulocytes for host defense.

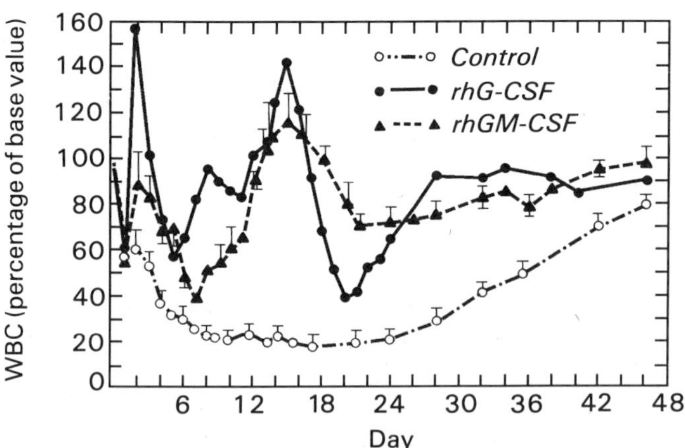

Figure 4. Recovery of peripheral white blood cells (WBC) after irradiation with 200-cGy total-body cobalt-60 and treatment with rhG-CSF (day 1 to day 15) and rhGM-CSF (day 1 to day 15). Data points are values (± SEM) representing 4 canines in the treatment groups and 10 canines in the control group.

Table 3. Antibiotic Therapy[1] for 350-cGy-Irradiated
Canines Treated With rhG-CSF or rhGM-CSF

Treatment	Time (days)
Control	16 (day 7 to day 22)
rhG-CSF	3 (day 11 to day 13)
rhGM-CSF	1 (day 6)

[1]Antibiotics were initiated when the white blood cell count
decreased below 1,000/mm³ and were continued until the
count increased above 1,000/mm³ for 3 consecutive days.

Administration of rhG-CSF or rhGM-CSF to 350-cGy-irradiated canines
resulted in a recovery pattern qualitatively similar to that seen for the sublethal
200-cGy-irradiated canines. The prompt release of reserve granulocytes was
followed by a decrease to leukocyte levels comparable to irradiated controls.
In the case of the 350-cGy-irradiated canines, the subsequent recovery phase
was delayed generally from day 12 to day 15, although leukocyte levels during
the nadir period were high enough (> 1,000/mm³) to decrease the number
of days the canines were on antibiotic therapy (table 3). Recovery, once initiated,

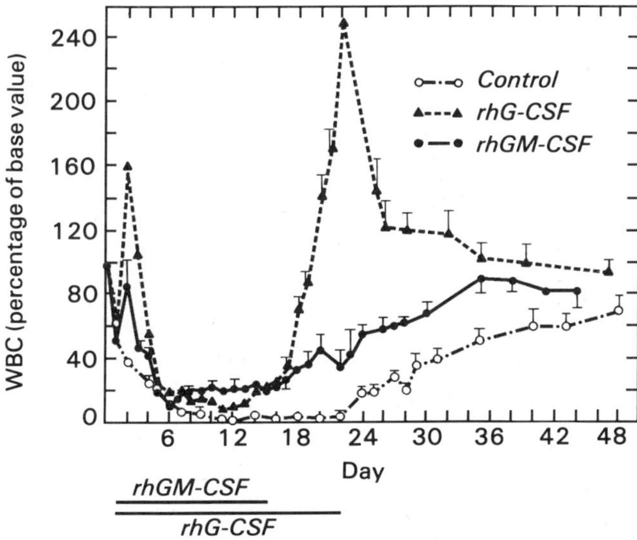

Figure 5. Recovery of peripheral white blood cells (WBC) after
irradiation with 350-cGy total-body cobalt-60 and treatment with
rhG-CSF (day 1 to day 21) and rhGM-CSF (day 1 to day 15). Data
points are values (± SEM) representing 4 canines in the treatment
groups and 12 canines in the control group.

Table 4. Lethality as a Function of Radiation Dose
and GM-CFC Survival and Its Modification by
Clinical Support and CSF Therapy

Radiation dose[1] (cGy)	Modification of lethality (percent)			GM-CFC survival (percent)
	Clinical support[2]			
	No	Yes	CSF therapy[3]	
200	0	ND	ND	8.0
260	50	0	ND	3.5
300	100	14	ND	2.0
340	100	50	ND	1.2
350	ND	60	0	1.0
400	ND	100	0	0.5
450	ND	ND	50	0.3
500	ND	ND	ND	0.1

ND, not done.
[1]Dose: cobalt-60; total-body, bilateral irradiation.
[2]Support: antibiotics, platelets, fluids, and nutrition.
[3]CSF: rhG-CSF, rhGM-CSF; D_0 73 cGy.

was evidenced by strong, consistent production of granulocytes during and after the treatment with recombinant CSF's. The differential production of granulocytes by rhG-CSF administered from day 1 through day 21 and rhGM-CSF injected from day 1 through day 15 is shown in figure 5. The additional 5 days of rhG-CSF treatment elicited an explosive production of granulocytes, while the shorter protocol of rhGM-CSF treatment appeared to establish a competent granulopoietic marrow capable of producing a sustained increased level of granulocytes. Both protocols resulted in 100-percent survival versus the 40-percent survival without CSF treatment.

Continuation of the recombinant CSF protocols (including increasing treatment through day 21 or day 24, depending on the radiation dose) has shown increased survival at radiation doses of 400 cGy and 450 cGy (table 4). Respective LD_{100} exposures were modified to 100-percent survival and 50-percent survival after irradiation with 400 cGy and 450 cGy with either rhG-CSF or rhGM-CSF therapy.

Discussion

These studies illustrate several key aspects about the therapeutic use of rhG-CSF and rhGM-CSF. These CSF's are effective in the canine as a preclinical model; they will decrease the severity and duration of neutropenia and, although unable to affect the severity of thrombocytopenia, will reduce its duration after sublethal and lethal radiation exposure. They will not exhaust the severely depleted stem cell population, and they will rescue lethally irradiated animals.

The high-dose lethal radiation models chosen were designed to reduce the stem cell and progenitor cell populations to levels that would not support survival in a percentage of animals irradiated. In fact, a key aspect of each lethal radiation model was the requirement for clinical support. Irradiation of canines or shielded monkeys without subsequent clinical support is always lethal. The use of fluids, antibiotics, and fresh irradiated platelets as substitution and replacement therapy significantly reduces the risks associated with infection from opportunistic pathogens and multiple points of hemorrhage.[43-45] Mean survival time of animals that did not survive increases from approximately 6 to 8 days, while support at the low lethal doses of radiation results in 100-percent survival. The key in therapeutic use of recombinant CSF's is the additional 6-8 days available to act on the recovering marrow hematopoietic precursors. It must be emphasized that the practical application of these concepts depends on the fact that damage to the stem cell system is reversible. The surviving fraction of hematopoietic stem cells must be capable of regeneration during the clinically manageable time period.

Available data indicate that the limiting factor in recovery from radiation-induced or drug-induced aplasia appears to be a lack of the appropriate CSF at the site of potential hematopoiesis.[19,24,31,37,38] The exogenous administration of rhG-CSF, rhGM-CSF, or interleukin-1 (IL-1) can override this limitation. The induction of recovery indicates that responsive target cells are available. The advantages of cytokine therapy are several (table 5), and all may be operative in these preclinical models. It is unknown whether other CSF's or interleukins are being produced *in situ*, within the marrow microenvironment. The radiosensitivity of environmental, stromal, or accessory cells relative to the induction and production of cytokines is unknown. It is possible that the therapeutic pharmacologic doses of rhG-CSF or rhGM-CSF are interacting with endogenous IL-1, IL-3, IL-6, and CSF's produced by the irradiated stromal cells *in situ*. There is increasing evidence that demonstrates *in vitro*[46-48] and *in vivo*[19,33,35,49,50] synergy between the interleukins and the CSF's.

The fraction of stem cells surviving in the 800-cGy-irradiated, shielded monkey was calculated to be approximately 0.0001,[37] whereas the fraction of stem cells surviving in the 350-cGy total-body-irradiated canine was approximately 0.01.[41,51] Our data show that survival is possible at these and lower levels of stem cell survival because the number of stem cells is above the threshold capable of self-renewal and because an adequate number of granulocyte lineage precursors capable of producing functional neutrophils are produced within the critical period of time required for competent host defense.

Table 5. Potential Advantageous Action of Cytokines at Several Levels in Modulation of Hematopoietic and Inflammatory Responses

Modulation level	Action
Bone marrow	Increase production of white cells and platelets. Stimulate production of CFC's, shorten G_0 period. Decrease maturation time.
Mature cells	Increase viability. Prime or activate neutrophils/macrophages. Stimulate release of cytokines.
Accessory cells	Stimulate release of cytokines in microenvironment/periphery.
Synergism	Increase hematopoiesis and production of mature cells.

The monkey model is of particular significance because it reveals the efficacy of a relatively short treatment protocol (7 consecutive days) on regeneration of a small number of surviving stem cells from a shielded area in an otherwise aplastic stem-cell-depleted marrow. As predicted,[6,8,10,11] the marrow regeneration began in the shielded but irradiated tibia and then progressed to the 800-cGy radiation-sterilized marrow of the iliac crest.[37] The canine model was used to further reduce the species-relative number of stem cells to result in 60-percent and 100-percent lethality. The use of rhGM-CSF and rhG-CSF was effective in promoting long-term survival through regeneration of granulocytes and platelets without promoting exhaustion of the irradiated and surviving stem cell population.

Therapeutic use of single-agent rhGM-CSF or rhG-CSF to promote regeneration of severely depleted stem cell and progenitor cell populations in otherwise lethally irradiated preclinical models without consequent exhaustion of the pluripotent stem cell pool is of particular significance in radiation accidents. The radiation exposure is usually ill defined and uncontrolled; therefore, bone marrow sparing is forecasted as a consequence of nonuniform and heterogeneous dose deposition.

Butturini et al.[52] have reported the advantageous use of rhGM-CSF in the Goiânia accident, and it has been reported that rhGM-CSF was used in the delayed treatment of the workers exposed to the cobalt-60 source in El Salvador. These data, combined with data from other preclinical models and many phase 1 and phase 2 clinical trials, support the use of rhGM-CSF or rhG-CSF in the treatment of radiation victims.[14,24,25,30-33,35-38]

Acknowledgment

We thank Dr. J. Sauber and Dr. R. Jackson for their surgical skill in implanting the minipumps, Dr. S. Stiefel for his pathological evaluations, and R. Brandenburg, L. Konradi, T. J. Lee, K. Noldy, and J. Hyde for their dedicated technical support. We are also indebted for the services and continued support of the AFRRI Radiation Sources Department and Information Services Department, and the expertise of Ms. G. Contreras.

References

1. Guskova, A. *Biomedical Section of the Soviet Report on Chernobyl, Appendix 7, Medical Biological Problems,* International Atomic Energy Agency (IAEA), Vienna, 1986.
2. Roberts, L. Radiation accident grips Goiânia. *Science* 238:1028-1031, 1989.
3. Baverstock, K. F., and Ash, P. J. N. O. A review of radiation accidents involving whole body exposure and the relevance to the $LD_{50/60}$ for man. *Br J Radiol* 56:837, 1983.
4. Cole, L. J., Haire, H. M., and Alpen, E. L. Partial shielding of dogs: Effectiveness of small external epicondylar lead cuffs against lethal x-radiation. *Radiat Res* 32:54-63, 1967.
5. Croizat, H., Frindel, E., and Tubiana, M. Abscopal effect of irradiation on haemopoietic stem cells of shielded bone marrow-role of migration. *Int J Radiat Biol* 30:347-358, 1976.
6. Gidali, J., and Lajtha, L. G. Regulation of hemopoietic stem cell turnover in partially irradiated mice. *Cell Tissue Kinet* 5:147-157, 1972.
7. Hansen, C. L., Michaelson, S. M., and Howland, J. W. Lethality of upper body exposure to x-radiation in beagles. *Public Health Rep* 76:242, 1961.
8. Knospe, W. H., Blom, J., and Crosby, W. H. Regeneration of locally irradiated bone marrow. I. Dose dependent, long-term changes in the rat, with particular emphasis upon vascular and stromal reaction. *Blood* 28:398-415, 1966.
9. Maillie, H. D., Krasavage, W., and Mermagen, H. On the partial body irradiation of the dog. *Health Phys* 12:833-837, 1966.
10. Maloney, M. A., and Patt, H. M. Migration of cells from shielded to irradiated marrow. *Blood* 39:804-808, 1972.
11. Nothdurft, W., Calvo, W., Klinnert, V., et al. Acute and long term alterations in the granulocyte/macrophage progenitor cell (GM-CFC) compartment of dogs after partial-body irradiation. *Int J Radiat Oncol Biol Phys* 12:949-957, 1986.
12. Broxmeyer, H. E., Williams, D. E., and Cooper, S. The influence *in vivo* of natural murine interleukin-3 on the proliferation of myeloid progenitor cells in mice recovering from sublethal dosages of cyclophosphamide. *Leuk Res* 11(2):201-205, 1987.
13. Cohen, A. M., Zsebo, K. M., Inoue, H., et al. *In vivo* stimulation of granulopoiesis by recombinant human granulocyte colony-stimulating factor. *Proc Natl Acad Sci USA* 84:2484-2488, 1987.
14. Fujisawa, M., Kobayashi, Y., Okabe, T., et al. Recombinant human granulocyte colony-stimulating factor induces granulocytosis *in vivo. Jpn J Cancer Res* 77:866-869, 1986.
15. Kindler, V., Thorens, B., deKossodo, S., et al. Stimulation of hematopoiesis *in vivo* by recombinant bacterial murine interleukin 3. *Proc Natl Acad Sci USA* 83:1001-1005, 1986.
16. Kobayashi, Y., Okabe, T., Urabe, A., et al. Human granulocyte colony stimulating factor produced by *Escherichia coli* shortens the period of granulocytopenia induced by irradiation in mice. *Jpn J Cancer Res* 78:763-770, 1987.
17. Lord, B. I., Molineux, G., Testa, N. G., et al. The kinetic response of haemopoietic precursors cells, *in vivo,* to highly purified, recombinant interleukin 3. *Lymphokine Res* 5:97-104, 1986.
18. Metcalf, D., Begley, C. G., Johnson, G. R., et al. Effects of purified bacterially synthesized murine multi-CSF (IL-3) on hematopoiesis in normal adult mice. *Blood* 68:46-57, 1986.
19. Moore, M. A. S., and Warren, D. J. Synergy of interleukin-1 and granulocyte colony stimulating factor: *In vivo* stimulation of stem cell recovery and hematopoietic regeneration following 5-fluorouracil treatment of mice. *Proc Natl Acad Sci USA* 84:7134-7138, 1987.

20. Morrissey, P., Charrier, K., Bressler, L., *et al.* The influence of IL-1 treatment on the reconstitution of the hematopoietic and immune systems after sublethal radiation. *J Immunol* 140:4204-4210, 1988.
21. Shimamura, M., Kobayashi, Y., Yuo, A., *et al.* Effect of human recombinant granulocyte colony-stimulating factor on hemopoietic injury in mice induced by 5-fluorouracil. *Blood* 69:353-355, 1987.
22. Stork, L., Barczuk, L., Kissinger, M., *et al.* Interleukin-1 accelerates murine granulocyte recovery following treatment with cyclophosphamide. *Blood* 73:938-944, 1989.
23. Tamura, M., Hattori, K., Nomura, H., *et al.* Induction of neutrophilic granulocytosis in mice by administration of purified human native granulocyte colony-stimulating factor (G-CSF). *Biochem Biophys Res Commun* 142:454-460, 1987.
24. Tanikawa, S., Nakao, I., Tsuneoka, K., *et al.* Effects of recombinant granulocyte colony stimulating factor (rG-CSF) and recombinant granulocyte-macrophage colony stimulating factor (rGM-CSF) on acute radiation hematopoietic injury in mice. *Exp Hematol* 17:883-888, 1989.
25. Lam, C., Mayer, P., Besemer, J., *et al.* Differential activation of dog, human, and monkey peripheral blood granulocytes by recombinant human granulocyte-macrophage colony-stimulating factor, *in vivo* hematopoietic activity in dogs. *J Cell Biochem [Suppl]* 13c:H401 (Abstract), 1989.
26. Lothrup, C. D., Jr., Warren, D. J., Souza, L. M., *et al.* Connection of canine cyclic hematopoiesis with recombinant human granulocyte colony stimulating factor. *Blood* 72:1324-1328, 1988.
27. MacVittie, T. J., D'Alesandro, M. M., Monroy, R. L., *et al.* Stimulation of hemopoiesis in the canine by *in vivo* administration of recombinant human GM-CSF (rhGM-CSF). *J Cell Biochem [Suppl]* 12A:152 (Abstract), 1988.
28. MacVittie, T. J., Schwartz, G. N., Monroy, R. L., *et al.* Stimulation of hemopoiesis in the canine by administration of recombinant human interleukin-1. *Exp Hematol* 16:537 (Abstract), 1988.
29. Schuening, F. G., Storb, R., Goehle, S., *et al.* Stimulation of canine hematopoiesis by recombinant human granulocyte-macrophage colony-stimulating factor. *Exp Hematol* 17:889-894, 1989.
30. Schuening, F. G., Storb, R., Goehle, S., *et al.* Effect of recombinant human granulocyte colony-stimulating factor on hematopoiesis of normal dogs and on hematopoietic recovery after otherwise lethal total-body irradiation. *Blood* 74:1308-1313, 1989.
31. MacVittie, T. J., Monroy, R. L., Patchen, M. L., *et al.* Therapeutic use of recombinant human G-CSF (rhG-CSF) in a canine model of sublethal and lethal whole-body irradiation. *Int J Radiat Biol* 57:723-736, 1990.
32. Donahue, R. E., Wang, E. A., Stone, D. K., *et al.* Stimulation of haematopoiesis in primates by continuous infusion of recombinant human GM-CSF. *Nature* 321:872-875, 1986.
33. Donahue, R. E., Seehra, J., Metzger, M., *et al.* Human IL-3 and GM-CSF act synergistically in stimulating hematopoiesis in primates. *Science* 241:1820-1823, 1988.
34. Gasparetto, C., Laver, J., Abboud, M., *et al.* Effects of interleukin-1 on hemopoietic progenitors: Evidence of stimulatory and inhibitory activities in a primate model. *Blood* 74:547-550, 1989.
35. Krumwieh, D., and Seiler, F. R. *In vivo* effects of recombinant colony stimulating factors on hematopoiesis in cynomolgus monkeys. *Transplant Proc* 21:2964-2967, 1989.
36. Mayer, P., Lam, C., Obenaus, H., *et al.* Recombinant human GM-CSF induces leukocytosis and activates peripheral blood polymorphonuclear neutrophils in non-human primates. *Blood* 70:206-213, 1987.
37. Monroy, R. L., Skelly, R. R., Taylor, P., *et al.* Recovery from severe hemopoietic suppression using recombinant human granulocyte-macrophage colony-stimulating factor. *Exp Hematol* 16:344-348, 1988.
38. Welte, K., Bonilla, M. A., Gillio, A. P., *et al.* Recombinant human granulocyte colony-stimulating factor: Effects on hematopoiesis in normal and cyclophosphamide-treated primates. *J Exp Med* 165:941-948, 1987.
39. Souza, L. M., Boone, T. C., Gabrilove, J., *et al.* Recombinant human granulocyte colony-stimulating factor: Effects on normal and leukemic myeloid cells. *Science* 232:61-65, 1986.
40. Monroy, R. L., MacVittie, T. J., Darden, J. H., *et al.* The rhesus monkey: A primate model for hemopoietic stem cell studies. *Exp Hematol* 14:904-911, 1986.

41. MacVittie, T. J., Monroy, R. L., Patchen, M. L., *et al.* Acute lethality and radiosensitivity of the canine hemopoietic system to cobalt-60 gamma and mixed neutron-gamma irradiation. In: *Response of Different Species to Total Body Irradiation.* J. J. Broerse and T. J. MacVittie, Eds. Martinus Nijhoff Publishers, Dordrecht, Netherlands, 1984, pp. 113-129.

42. Broerse, J. J., van Bekkum, D. W., Hollander, C. F., *et al.* Mortality of monkeys after exposure to fission neutrons and the effect of autologous bone marrow transplantation. *Int J Radiat Biol* 34:253-264, 1978.

43. Jackson, D. P., Sorenson, D. K., Cronkite, E. P., *et al.* Effectiveness of transfusion of fresh and lyophilized platelets in controlling bleeding due to thrombocytopenia. *J Clin Invest* 38:1689-1697, 1959.

44. Perman, V., Cronkite, E. P., Bond, V. P., *et al.* The regenerative ability of hemopoietic tissue following lethal x-irradiation in dogs. *Blood* 19:724-737, 1962.

45. Sorenson, D. K., Bond, V. P., Cronkite, E. P., *et al.* An effective therapeutic regimen for the hemopoietic phase of the acute radiation syndrome in dogs. *Radiat Res* 13:669-676, 1960.

46. Ferrero, D., Tarella, C., Badoni, R., *et al.* Granulocyte-macrophage colony-stimulating factor requires interaction with accessory cells or granulocyte colony-stimulating factor for full stimulation of human myeloid progenitors. *Blood* 73:402-405, 1989.

47. McNiece, I. K., Andrews, R., Stewart, M., *et al.* Action of interleukin-3, G-CSF, and GM-CSF on highly enriched human hematopoietic progenitor cells: Synergistic interaction of GM-CSF plus G-CSF. *Blood* 74:110-114, 1989.

48. Ikebuchi, K., Clark, S. C., Ihle, J. N., *et al.* Granulocyte colony-stimulating factor enhances interleukin 3-dependent proliferation of multipotential hemopoietic progenitors. *Proc Natl Acad Sci USA* 85:3445-3450, 1988.

49. Broxmeyer, H. E., Williams, D. E., Hangoc, G., *et al.* Synergistic myelopoietic actions *in vivo* after administration to mice of combinations of purified natural murine colony-stimulating factor 1, recombinant murine interleukin 3, and recombinant murine granulocyte/macrophage colony-stimulating factor. *Proc Natl Acad Sci USA* 84:3871-3875, 1987.

50. Williams, D. E., Hangoc, G., Cooper, S., *et al.* The effects of purified recombinant murine interleukin-3 and/or purified natural murine CSF-1 *in vivo* on the proliferation of murine high- and low-proliferative potential colony-forming cells: Demonstration of *in vivo* synergism. *Blood* 70(2):401-403, 1987.

51. Vriesendorp, H. M., and van Bekkum, D. W. Susceptibility to total body irradiation. In: *Response of Different Species to Total Body Irradiation.* J. J. Broerse and T. J. MacVittie, Eds. Martinus Nijhoff Publishers, Dordrecht, Netherlands, 1984, pp. 43-57.

52. Butturini, A., DeSouza, P. C., Gale, R. P., *et al.* Use of recombinant granulocyte-macrophage colony stimulating factor in the Brazil radiation accident. *Lancet* II:471-475, 1988.

Myeloprotective Effects of Interleukin-1 Following Exposure to Chemoradiotherapy

Joseph Laver, Alfred Gillio, Miguel Abboud,
Cristina Gasparetto, David Warren,
Richard J. O'Reilly,
and Malcolm A. S. Moore

Introduction

Interleukin-1 (IL-1), a cytokine with multiple immunological and inflammatory functions, has recently been demonstrated to play a role in hematopoietic regulation.[1] Although IL-1 alone does not stimulate hematopoietic colony growth, it is synergistic with other growth factors and has been shown to be identical to hematopoietin-1.[2] In addition to having a direct effect on early hematopoietic progenitors, IL-1 is capable of inducing production of various colony-stimulating factors (CSF's) by accessory cell populations in the hematopoietic tissue.[3] Administering IL-1 to mice pretreated with chemotherapy accelerated hematopoietic recovery and reduced the nadir in neutrophil count.[4] Administering IL-1 to mice before or shortly after lethal irradiation protected them from severe neutropenia and subsequent death from septicemia.[5,6] These results suggest that IL-1 induces a chain of events that probably affects the radiosensitivity of early hematopoietic progenitors.[7] The effects of IL-1 on hematopoietic recovery after chemotherapy, together with IL-1's radioprotective effect, indicate that this cytokine might have therapeutic potential when given either alone or in combination with other CSF's in the treatment of chemoradiotherapy-induced myelosuppression. In contrast to stimulating blood-forming cells, IL-1 may induce endogenous production of hematopoietic inhibitors, including various prostaglandins, tumor necrosis factor alpha (TNFα), and interferon-gamma.[8,9] Thus, the *in vivo* hematopoietic effects of IL-1 depend on the balance between its stimulatory and inhibitory activities.

J. LAVER*, A. GILLIO, M. ABBOUD, C. GASPARETTO, D. WARREN, R. J. O'REILLY, and M. A. S. MOORE, Bone Marrow Transplantation Service, and The James Ewing Laboratory of Developmental Hematopoiesis, Memorial Sloan-Kettering Cancer Center, New York, New York 10021.

*Current address: Department of Pediatrics, Medical University of South Carolina, 171 Ashley Avenue, Charleston, South Carolina 29425.

Treatment of Radiation Injuries, Edited by
D. Browne *et al.*, Plenum Press, New York, 1990

This chapter summarizes data from our murine, primate, and human studies of the effects of IL-1 on the recovery of hematopoietic cells after myelosuppressive chemotherapy and radiation.

Materials and Methods

In vitro and *in vivo* procedures for studying IL-1 effects in murine, primate, and human systems are described below.

Hematopoietic Growth Factors

Recombinant human IL-1 alpha (rhIL-1α) and beta (rhIL-1β) were obtained from Syntex, Palo Alto, CA. Mice were injected with rhIL-1α at 0.2 μg/dose once or twice daily. Primates were injected with 1 μg/kg of rhIL-1β daily as described below. *In vitro* cultures were done with marrow cells in the presence of recombinant human granulocyte CSF (rhG-CSF; Amgen, Thousand Oaks, CA), recombinant human granulocyte-macrophage CSF (rhGM-CSF; Amgen, Thousand Oaks, CA), or rhIL-3 (Immunex, Seattle, WA).

Mice

C3H/HeJ mice were used for the *in vivo* studies of IL-1 in animals treated with 150 mg/kg of 5-fluorouracil (5-FU). BALB/c mice were used to study the effects of IL-1 on irradiated animals.

Primates

Cynomolgus monkeys *(Macaca fasicularis)* were used in this study. Animals were treated with 150 mg/kg of 5-FU (75 mg/kg/day for 2 days) and then with 1 μg/kg/day of IL-1 for 2 days, 7 days, or 14 days. Primates undergoing marrow transplantation received 1,000 cGy followed by infusion of 7.5 x 10^8 marrow cells and 1 μg/kg/day of rhIL-1β for 7 days. Daily blood counts and weekly marrow aspirates were done to assess the effects of IL-1. Primate whole blood was collected every 3 days and immediately placed on ice, and the serum was separated and frozen at -80°C.

Granulocyte-Macrophage Colony-Forming Unit

Bone marrow cells obtained from humans and primates were separated by Ficoll-Hypaque and 3-percent gelatin, respectively. Low-density cells were washed and resuspended in Iscove's modified Dulbecco's medium (IMDM; Gibco, Grand Island, NY) supplemented with 20-percent fetal calf serum (FCS; Hyclone, Logan, UT). The granulocyte-macrophage colony-forming units (GM-CFU's) were prepared as previously described.[10] Briefly, cells were plated at a concentration of 1 x 10^5/mL in 35-mm tissue culture dishes containing 1-mL mixtures of 0.36-percent Agarose (FMS, Rockland, ME) and 20-percent FCS in the presence of rhG-CSF (1,000 U/mL), rhGM-CSF (1,000 U/mL), and rhIL-3 (50 ng/mL).

Cocultivation Assay

To investigate whether administering rhIL-1β could induce hematopoietic inhibitory effects, we cultured normal primate marrow cells with sera obtained from primates receiving rhIL-1β. The serum-free medium was prepared as previously described.[11] The final concentration of the mixture contained bovine serum albumin (30 mg/mL), cholesterol (5 μg/mL), low-density lipoprotein (50 μg/mL), iron-saturated human transferrin (300 μg/mL), and calcium chloride (90 μg/mL) (Sigma Chemicals, St. Louis, MO). Exogenous stimuli for colony growth included 10-percent serum-free conditioned medium 5637, 1,000 U/mL of rhG-CSF, or 1,000 U/mL of GM-CSF. Cultures were incubated at 37°C in humidified 5-percent CO_2 in air, and GM-CFU colonies were scored on day 7 and day 14.

Human Marrow Cells

Bone marrow cells were obtained from normal healthy volunteers who gave informed consent. Marrow buffy coat cells were collected and then separated by neutral density centrifugation (Ficoll-Hypaque), and subsequently subjected to two cycles of adherence. Low-density cells were then prepared for culture in a delta assay, which assesses early hematopoietic progenitors (figure 1). Cells

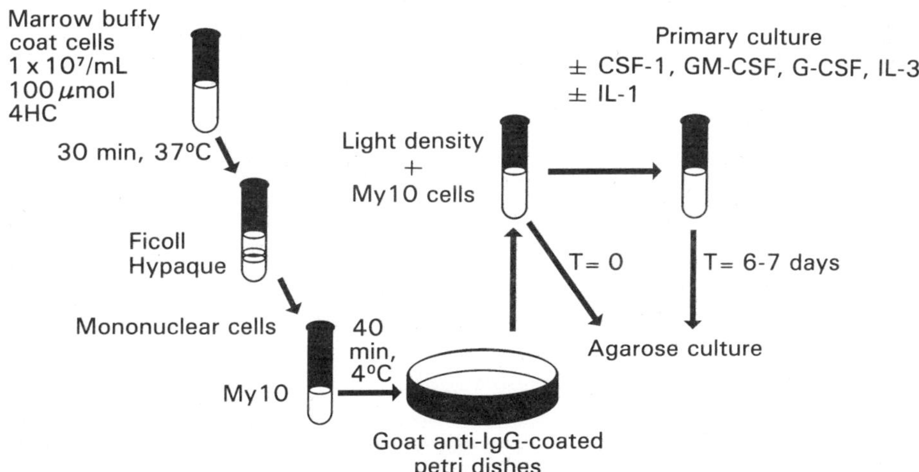

Figure 1. Diagram of the delta assay. Following 4HC purging and CD34-positive selection, human cells are plated for GM-CFU (input). Simultaneously, cells are cultured in a liquid phase in the presence of various hematopoietic growth factors or their combinations for 7 days. The cells are replated in a GM-CFU assay with various growth factors (output). The difference between output and input (the delta) reflects the presence of pre-CFU populations.

were exposed to 100 μmol of 4-hydroperoxycyclophosphamide (4HC) for 30 minutes and then mixed with a monoclonal antibody directed against the CD34 antigen. Subsequently, CD34-positive cells were selected by means of the antibody-mediated-plate-binding technique (panning). These cells were enriched for hematopoietic progenitors with a diminished frequency of committed progenitors and accessory cells. CD34-positive cells were cultured in semisolid clonogenic assays for GM-CFU in the presence of different CSF's: rhG-CSF, rhGM-CSF, or rhIL-3 with or without rhIL-1β. In parallel, cells were cultured in a liquid phase in the presence of rhG-CSF, rhGM-CSF, or rhIL-3 with or without IL-1 in IMDM supplemented with 20-percent FCS. After 7 days in culture, cells were replated in semisolid assays in the presence of rhCSF's with or without rhIL-1β. The recovery value of colonies after 7 days of suspension was compared to input, and the increase in the colony number reflected the presence of pre-CFU progenitors. In a set of experiments designed to assess the radioprotective effects of IL-1 on these progenitors, cells were irradiated before culture, and survival curves were constructed for clonogenic cells. The effects of IL-1 on the radiosensitivity of pre-CFU progenitors were assessed by comparing colony output in secondary cultures in the presence and absence of rhIL-1β.

Serum Levels of TNFα

An ELISA (Endogen, Inc., Boston, MA) specific for TNFα (no cross-reaction with other cytokines such as TNFβ, rhIL-1, rhIL-2, or rhIL-6) was used to measure TNFα in sera of primates receiving rhIL-1β. Absorbance at 405 nm was determined on an automated ELISA reader (Biotek, Inc., Berlington, VA) as directed. The test sensitivity was 10 pg/mL.

Results

The effects of IL-1 on the recovery of hematopoietic cells after myelosuppressive chemotherapy and radiation in our studies are summarized below.

In Vivo Murine Studies

C3H/HeJ mice treated with 150 mg/kg of 5-FU exhibited neutropenia for 14 days. Mice given rhG-CSF for 14 days (2 μg twice daily) had restored neutrophil counts at normal values 5 days earlier than mice that did not receive the factor, but the animals were profoundly neutropenic for 9 days. A 0.2-μg/dose of rhIL-1α given after chemotherapy for 4-10 days twice daily reduced the neutrophil nadir and accelerated recovery to a greater extent than was observed with rhG-CSF alone (animals were neutropenic for 6 days). The combination of rhG-CSF and rhIL-1α administered after 5-FU therapy resulted in accelerated neutrophil recovery, although the results were additive rather than synergistic. Giving rhIL-1α 24 hours before 5-FU was counterproductive and resulted in a delay in recovery of neutrophils.

Table 1. Survival of BALB/c Mice Receiving 850 cGy Total-Body Irradiation in Combination With rhIL-1α or rhG-CSF

Treatment[1]		Survival
Before irradiation	After irradiation	Number/Sample
None	None	0/10
rhG-CSF	None	0/10
None	rhG-CSF	5/7
rhG-CSF	rhG-CSF	0/5
rhIL-1α	None	10/10
rhIL-1α	rhG-CSF	10/10

[1]Mice were given 2 μg of rhG-CSF intraperitoneally (i.p.) 20 hours before irradiation or twice daily for 14 days after irradiation. The 0.2-μg dose of rhIL-1α was injected i.p. 20 hours before irradiation.

The radioprotective properties of rhIL-1α were studied in BALB/c mice, which are particularly susceptible to the effects of radiation. A 0.2-μg dose of rhIL-1α administered 20 hours before 850 cGy total-body irradiation prevented what would otherwise have been 100-percent mortality by day 14 (table 1). Injection of rhIL-1α after irradiation, either alone or in combination with rhG-CSF, was also significantly radioprotective. Administration of rhG-CSF before irradiation was not radioprotective—all mice died after 850-cGy irradiation. After 750-cGy irradiation, only 20 percent of the animals survived for 14 days. Administration

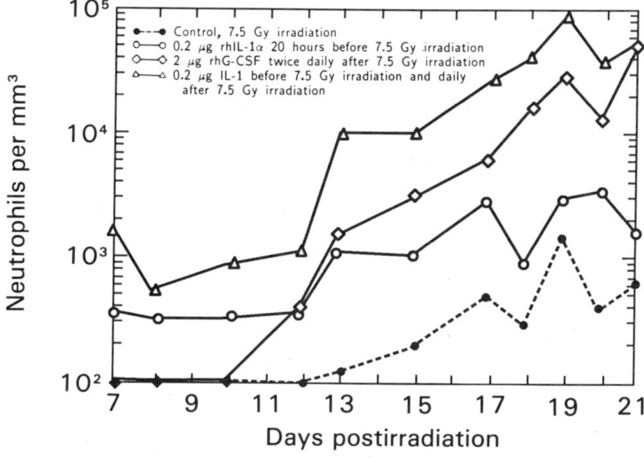

Figure 2. Effect of rhIL-1α and rhG-CSF on neutrophil recovery in irradiated BALB/c mice.

of rhIL-1α before irradiation accelerated the neutrophil recovery significantly and increased survival to 100 percent. Giving rhIL-1α before irradiation and rhG-CSF after irradiation proved to be synergistic; the increase in neutrophil count was up to tenfold greater, and the neutrophil nadir was abolished (figure 2).

In Vivo and In Vitro Primate Studies

In primates, administration of 150 mg/kg of 5-FU resulted in profound neutropenia, lasting for 30 days. Administration of rhIL-1β at 1 μg/kg/day for 2 days or 7 days shortened the period of neutropenia to 17 days. Administration of rhIL-1β at the same dose for 14 days resulted in relatively delayed recovery (table 2). *In vitro* studies showed that 2 days and 7 days of IL-1 therapy resulted in significantly increased frequency of marrow progenitors responding to rhG-CSF, rhGM-CSF, and rhIL-3 by day 14 after 5-FU therapy (figure 3). Animals treated for 14 days with IL-1 had a low frequency of progenitors on day 14 but recovered by day 21 (7 days after cessation of IL-1 therapy). To further investigate the delayed recovery of progenitors in animals receiving the 14-day course, we cocultured normal monkey marrow with sera that had been obtained on different days after 5-FU therapy. On day 9 after 5-FU, an inhibitory activity was detected in sera of animals treated with rhIL-1β for 14 days. The inhibition was reversible with the addition of anti-TNFα monoclonal antibody. The serum level of TNFα corresponding with the inhibitory activity was 918 pg/mL (in controls and animals treated for 2 days or 7 days the level was undetectable).

In another set of experiments, animals that received 1,000 cGy total-body irradiation were given marrow grafts with or without rhIL-1β (rhIL-1β was given at 1 μg/kg/day for 7 days after marrow transplantation). Compared to controls, animals treated with rhIL-1β did not show accelerated marrow progenitor frequency or neutrophil recovery.

Table 2. Neutrophil Recovery in Primates
Treated With rhIL-1β After Administration of 5-Fluorouracil

Treatment	Neutrophil recovery[1] (days)
Control	30
rhIL-1β:	
2 days	17
7 days	17
14 days	23

[1]Neutrophils > 500/mm^3.

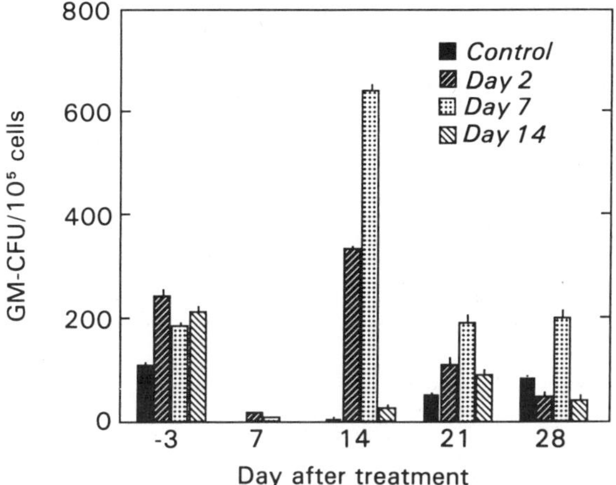

Figure 3. Progenitor recovery in primates treated with 5-fluorouracil. GM-CFU frequency in recipients of rhIL-1β for 2 days or 7 days occurred earlier and at higher magnitude than in primates treated for 14 days or in untreated controls.

In Vitro Human Studies

Radiation survival curves of CD34-positive marrow cells were constructed in the presence of rhG-CSF, rhGM-CSF, and rhIL-3 (each of them with and without rhIL-1β). Table 3 shows D_0 (the radiation dose reducing survival to 37 percent of an initial value on the straight portion of the survival curve) calculated for each cytokine. The presence of rhIL-1β in culture resulted in a significant increase of D_0's in GM-CFU's. In addition to its radioprotective

Table 3. D_0's of Human GM-CFU in the Presence of Various Growth Factors With or Without RhIL-1β

Treatment	D_0 (cGy)[1]		
	rhG-CSF	rhGM-CSF	rhIL-3
Without rhIL-1β	103	127	116
With rhIL-1 β	205	205	215

[1]D_0, radiation dose that reduces survival to 37 percent of an initial value on the straight portion of the survival curve.

Table 4. Change in Human GM-CFU Frequency
in a Two-Step (Delta) Assay Following
In Vitro Irradiation[1]

Radiation dose (cGy)	Fold increase compared to GM-CFU on day 0	
	Without rhIL-1β	With rhIL-1β
0	3.30	6.04
100	0.30	3.30
200	0	2.80

[1]After *in vitro* irradiation, cells were put in liquid phase with rhIL-3, with or without rhIL-1β.

effects on committed hematopoietic progenitors, rhIL-1β had similar effects on early hematopoietic progenitors. Employing a two-step culture assay (delta assay), we were able to demonstrate that the presence of rhIL-1β in culture resulted in a fivefold relative increase in the survival of pre-CFU progenitors (table 4). Adding the rhIL-1β to cultures after irradiation did not result in a radioprotective effect.

Discussion

IL-1 has been recognized to be a cytokine with immunomediating, inflammatory, and hematopoietic effects. In the hematopoietic system, IL-1's dual activity is demonstrated by having a direct effect on stem cells and by inducing production of other growth factors. The therapeutic potential of IL-1 alone or in combination with other CSF's has been under investigation recently. Our study shows that in mice, rhIL-1α alone or combined with other CSF's can shorten the period of neutropenia and decrease the nadir in neutrophil count after chemoradiotherapy. Other investigators have reported similar effects when IL-1 was administered to mice receiving radiation or chemotherapy.[4,5,6]

In primates, giving rhIL-1β for 2 days or 7 days after 5-FU therapy resulted in accelerated recovery of neutrophils compared to controls. Although severe neutropenia was shortened, it was still observed for more than 2 weeks (in controls, for 4 weeks). Prolonged administration of rhIL-1β to monkeys was counterproductive because it induced the production of hematopoietic inhibitors such as TNFα. Therefore, the therapeutic use of IL-1 in enhancing hematological recovery after myelosuppressive therapy depends on the balance between its stimulatory and inhibitory activities. Our data indicate that short courses of IL-1 are myelostimulatory, whereas prolonged administration is less effective.[12] When rhIL-1β was given to monkeys after bone marrow transplantation, accelerated hematopoietic reconstitution did not result. The difference in response to IL-1 after chemotherapy and marrow transplantation might be explained by the need for additional factors to promote engraftment of cells responsible for hematopoietic reconstitution. Data generated in mice support this concept. Administration of IL-1 combined with different CSF's might result in rapid hematopoietic recovery after bone marrow transplantation.

The radioprotective effects of IL-1 when administered before or after radiation raised the question of whether IL-1 has a direct effect on survival of progenitors or acts through the production of other cytokines by the accessory cells. Moreb et al.[13] demonstrated that IL-1 induced a chemoprotective effect on hematopoietic progenitors *in vitro*. In our study, the effects in the delta assay indicate that IL-1 has a direct radioprotective effect on early marrow progenitors, but other mechanisms involving accessory cells are also probably in effect *in vivo*.

In conclusion, our results show that IL-1 can accelerate hematopoietic recovery after chemoradiotherapy, and is radioprotective when administered before or close to the time of radiation. However, further studies are needed to assess the potential role IL-1 might play in the treatment of humans with radiation injuries.

Acknowledgment

This work was supported by public service grants CA-32516, CA-20194, and CA-23766 from the National Cancer Institute; American Cancer Society Grant CH-3k, the Gar-Reichman Fund of the Cancer Research Institute; and a Syntex Corporation grant. C. Gasparetto is supported by the Italian Association for Cancer Research.

References

1. Moore, M. A. S., and Warren, D. J. Interleukin-1 and G-CSF synergism: *In vivo* stimulation of stem cell recovery and hematopoietic regeneration following 5-fluorouracil treatment in mice. *Proc Natl Acad Sci USA* 84:7134-7138, 1987.
2. Jubinsky, P. I., and Stanley, E. R. Purification of hematopoietin-1: A multilineage hematopoietic growth factor. *Proc Natl Acad Sci USA* 82:2764-2767, 1985.
3. Bagby, G. C., Dinarello, C. A., and Wallace, P. Interleukin-1 stimulates granulocyte-macrophage colony-stimulating activity release by vascular endothelial cells. *J Clin Invest* 78:1316-1320, 1986.
4. Stork, L., Barczuk, L., Kissinger, M., et al. Interleukin-1 accelerates murine granulocytes following treatment with cyclophosphamide. *Blood* 73:938-944, 1989.
5. Neta, R., and Oppenheim, J. J. Cytokines in therapy of radiation injury. *Blood* 72:1093-1095, 1988.
6. Neta, R., Douches, S. D., and Oppenheim, J. J. Interleukin 1 is a radioprotector. *J Immunol* 136:2483-2485, 1986.

7. Neta, R., Sztein, M. B., Oppenheim, J. J., et al. The *in vivo* effects of interleukin 1. I. Bone marrow cells are induced to cycle after administration of interleukin 1. *J Immunol* 139:1861-1866, 1987.
8. Broxmeyer, H. E. Biomolecule-cell interactions and the regulation of myelopoiesis. *Int J Cell Cloning* 4:378-389, 1986.
9. Zucali, J. R., Dinarello, C. A., Oblon, D. J., et al. Interleukin-1 stimulates fibroblasts to produce granulocyte-macrophage colony-stimulating activity and prostaglandin E_2. *J Clin Invest* 77:1857-1863, 1986.
10. Laver, J., Ebell, W., and Castro-Malaspina, H. Radiobiological properties of the human hematopoietic microenvironment: Contrasting sensitivities of proliferative capacity and hematopoietic function to *in vitro* irradiation. *Blood* 67:1090-1097, 1986.
11. Iscove, N. N., Guilbert, L. J., and Weyman, C. Complete replacement of serum in primary cultures of erythropoietin-dependent red cell precursors (CFU-E) by albumin, transferrin, iron, unsaturated fatty acids, lecithin, and cholesterol. *Exp Cell Res* 126:121-127, 1980.
12. Gasparetto, C., Laver, J., Abboud, M., et al. Effects of interleukin-1 on hematopoietic progenitors: Evidence of stimulatory and inhibitory activities in a primate model. *Blood* 74:547-550, 1989.
13. Moreb, J., Zucali, J. R., Gross, M. A., et al. Protective effects of IL-1 on human hematopoietic progenitor cells treated *in vitro* with 4-hydroperoxycyclophosphamide. *J Immunol* 142:1937-1942, 1989.

Effects of Combined Application of IL-3 and G-CSF on Subhuman Primates

Dorothee Krumwieh, Ernst Weinmann, Bernhard Siebold, and Friedrich R. Seiler

Introduction

In vitro proliferation, differentiation, and functional activation of hematopoietic progenitor cells are regulated by colony-stimulating factors (CSF's). The four major recombinant human CSF's—interleukin-3 (IL-3), granulocyte-macrophage CSF (GM-CSF), granulocyte CSF (G-CSF), and megakaryocyte CSF—have been characterized as mainly responsible for the process whereby bone marrow progenitors mature into granulocytes and macrophages.[1] Recent progress in molecular cloning of human and murine genes for these hematopoietic growth and differentiation factors has provided large amounts of highly purified recombinant glycoproteins.[2-5] All four factors are also being investigated for their clinical efficacy in alleviating various insufficiencies of the blood-cell-forming system.[6-8]

In vitro studies have already shown that combinations of different CSF's exhibit additive or even synergistic effects.[9,10] Consecutive treatment of macaques with IL-3 and GM-CSF has shown that IL-3 enhances the number of GM-CSF-responsive bone marrow progenitors, thus reducing the amount of GM-CSF required for a desired response.[11-13]

We investigated the effects of the combination of IL-3 and G-CSF on the stimulation of hematopoiesis in normal cynomolgus monkeys; in particular, we compared simultaneous and sequential application schemes.

Materials and Methods

Cynomolgus monkeys (*Macaca fascicularis*), each weighing 2-3 kg, were obtained from our animal-breeding facility. The monkeys were individually

D. KRUMWIEH, E. WEINMANN, B. SIEBOLD, and F. R. SEILER, Research Laboratories, Behringwerke AG, P.O. Box 1140, D-3550 Marburg/Lahn, Federal Republic of Germany.

Treatment of Radiation Injuries, Edited by
D. Browne *et al.,* Plenum Press, New York, 1990

housed in stainless steel cages, and food and tap water were available *ad libitum.*
The animals were anesthetized with ketamine hydrochloride (Parke-Davis,
Munich, FRG).

The rhIL-3 cDNA was cloned from peripheral blood leukocytes, and the
gene product was expressed in yeast. The molecular weight was 14-18 kDa,
and the specific biological activity was above 1 x 10^7 U/mg of glycoprotein,
as determined in the human bone marrow cell-proliferation assay. The rhG-
CSF cDNA was obtained from human bladder tumor 5637 cells, and the gene
product was also expressed in yeast. The highly purified glycoprotein had a
molecular weight of 18 kDa and a biological activity of about 5 x 10^7 U/mg
protein. All preparations used were free of detectable endotoxin (10 pg/10
μg protein) as determined by Limulus Lysate Assay (Pyroquant, Walldorf, FRG).

Cynomolgus monkeys were treated with IL-3 and G-CSF applied sequentially
as follows: rhIL-3 (10 μg/kg/day and 100 μg/kg/day) was administered on 8
consecutive days followed by rhG-CSF (10 μg/kg/day) for 8 consecutive days.
For the reverse application, rhG-CSF (100 μg/kg/day) was injected on 5
consecutive days followed by rhIL-3 (100 μg/kg/day and 10 μg/kg/day) for
10 consecutive days. In the last set of experiments, G-CSF (100 μg/kg/day and
10 μg/kg/day) and IL-3 (10 μg/kg/day) were injected simultaneously at different
injection sites for 26 consecutive days. All injections were applied as an
intravenous bolus in a volume of 2 mL/kg/body weight. Growth factors were
diluted in 0.9 percent sodium chloride containing 2 percent human serum
albumin. Blood samples were drawn before CSF's were administered. Every
2 days, 2 mL of blood were collected in EDTA-coated tubes starting on day -4.
Hematological examinations included total white blood cell counts and
differentiation (Pappenheim stain), platelet counts (Coulter Electronics, Krefeld,
FRG), reticulocyte number (brilliant cresyl blue stain), hemoglobin, and
hematocrit (Boehringer, Mannheim, FRG).

Results

RhIL-3 and rhG-CSF were administered in different schedules to determine
whether their actions were additive or synergistic. The administration schedule
greatly influenced the efficacy of both factors, as demonstrated in the changes
of the peripheral white blood cell count (figure 1). For the sequential
combination of IL-3 followed by G-CSF, a suboptimal dosage of G-CSF (10
μg/kg/day) was combined with 10 μg/kg/day or 100 μg/kg/day of pretreatment
phase with IL-3. This schedule resulted in a dose-dependent synergistic effect
of IL-3 enhancing the G-CSF response. The differential counts showed an
increase mainly in segmented neutrophils and bands. No changes were
observed in monocytes, eosinophils, and basophils. Only the animals treated
with IL-3 at 100 μg/kg/day showed a rise in platelet counts (table 1).

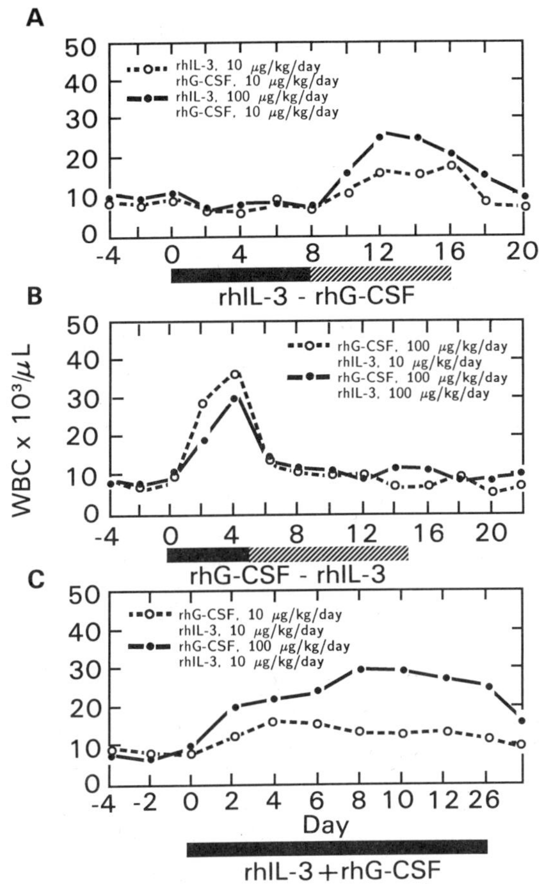

Figure 1. (A) Effect of sequential IL-3 and G-CSF treatment in monkeys on peripheral blood cell formation. IL-3 (10 μg/kg/day or 100 μg/kg/day) was injected on day 1 through day 8 followed by G-CSF (10 μg/kg/day) on day 9 through day 16. (B) Effect of reversed application of IL-3 and G-CSF on hematopoiesis of monkeys. G-CSF (100 μg/kg/day) was administered through day 5, followed by IL-3 (10 μg/kg/day or 100 μg/kg/day) on day 6 through day 15. (C) Effect of simultaneous application of G-CSF (10 μg/kg/day or 100 μg/kg/day) and IL-3 (10 μg/kg/day) for 26 consecutive days. (A), (B), and (C) show total white blood cell (WBC) count x 10³ μL for two separate monkeys.

The reverse experiment was performed using G-CSF in a known effective dosage (100 μg/kg/day) followed by IL-3 (10 μg/kg/day or 100 μg/kg/day) to examine the influence of the order of sequential application. At the end of the G-CSF administration phase, the data showed that white blood cell levels dropped to starting values, despite continued administration of IL-3. IL-3 was not able to either enhance the primary G-CSF response or to prolong its efficacy phase. The increase in white blood cell counts under G-CSF administration was due to rising neutrophil counts only. However, the reverse application schedule brought about a pronounced increase in platelet counts in all treated animals.

A third set of experiments was performed to determine the effects of simultaneous application of IL-3 and G-CSF and to compare the results to the effects of sequential application. Over a treatment period of 26 consecutive days, administering both IL-3 and G-CSF at 10 μg/kg/day did not produce any changes in the peripheral white blood cell count, even when in another

Table 1. Effects of Colony-Stimulating Factors on Platelet Counts[1] of Cynomolgus Monkeys

Day	Colony-stimulating factors					
	rhIL-3 and rhG-CSF[2]	rhIL-3 and rhG-CSF[3]	rhG-CSF and rhIL-3[4]	rhG-CSF and rhIL-3[5]	rhG-CSF and rhIL-3[6]	rhG-CSF and rhIL-3[7]
-4	319± 33	343± 7	391± 1	362± 26	357± 57	379± 44
-2	327± 44	363± 35	322± 28	342± 1	326± 51	348± 20
0	267± 29	416± 6	377± 23	349± 4	356± 1	418±103
2	250± 13	469± 93	361± 36	368± 10	386± 24	376±134
4	271± 44	482± 61	378± 1	393± 0	414± 49	332±163
6	277± 24	519± 9	306± 10	343± 16	293±151	311±227
8	280± 47	555± 21	248± 10	344± 12	397± 26	447± 6
10	278± 66	546± 16	320± 6	412± 54	362± 21	384± 18
12	303± 37	538± 3	426± 9	535± 43	407± 19	288± 91
14	279± 21	519± 10	607± 26	615± 47	(8)	(8)
16	286± 7	498± 37	627± 60	741± 45	(8)	(8)
18	295± 0	461± 88	532± 47	650± 40	(8)	(8)
20	301±18	504± 69	460± 5	623± 67	(8)	(8)
22	(8)	(8)	457± 2	612± 79	(8)	(8)
26	(8)	(8)	(8)	(8)	345± 29	482± 20
28	(8)	(8)	(8)	(8)	363± 28	520± 66

[1] x 10[3]

[2] Injections of rhIL-3 (10 μg/kg/day) on day 1 through day 8 followed by rhG-CSF (10 μg/kg/day) on day 9 through day 16.
[3] Injections of rhIL-3 (100 μg/kg/day) on day 1 through day 8 followed by rhG-CSF (10 μg/kg/day) on day 9 through day 16.
[4] Injections of rhG-CSF (100 μg/kg/day) on day 1 through day 5 followed by rhIL-3 (10 μg/kg/day) on day 6 through day 15.
[5] Injections of rhG-CSF (100 μg/kg/day) on day 1 through day 5 followed by rhIL-3 (100 μg/kg/day) on day 6 through day 15.
[6] Injections of rhG-CSF (10 μg/kg/day) and rhIL-3 (10 μg/kg/day) simultaneously at different injection sites on day 1 through day 26.
[7] Injections of rhG-CSF (100 μg/kg/day) and rhIL-3 (10 μg/kg/day) simultaneously at different injection sites on day 1 through day 26.
[8] No data.

experiment the dose of G-CSF was increased to 100 μg/kg/day for the same administration time. Only the increase in neutrophils that can be reached using G-CSF alone at those dose levels was observed. Again, no changes in the other myeloid lineages could be detected. Furthermore, no platelet induction could be seen. The animals showed a modest fall in hemoglobin of 1.8 g/dL to 2.0 g/dL at the end of the study. These data were correlated with the slight drop in hematocrit.

Discussion

To determine the synergistic capacity of IL-3 in combination with G-CSF, we compared different application schedules for both factors and their synergistic action. The sequential application of IL-3 followed by G-CSF resulted in an increase in neutrophils. The concept of receptor-mediated events with a subsequent modification of the responsiveness of the cells to the various CSF's has been reported for the murine system,[14] and might be a possible reason for the synergistic action. The loss of IL-3 responsiveness with the maturation of neutrophils has recently been reported for human and murine bone-marrow-derived cells.[15] These observations could help explain the absence of the normally enhancing and stimulatory effect of IL-3 on the number of circulating neutrophils seen when the order of administration is reversed. However, the capacity of IL-3 to stimulate megakaryocyte progenitors was unaffected by this schedule. The possible effect of G-CSF in triggering stem cells in G_0 to begin cell cycling is under intensive investigation.[10] Such a function of G-CSF could possibly explain our results. The synergistic action of IL-3 and GM-CSF or G-CSF[9] seems to play a role in regulating normal hematopoiesis *in vivo*. More intensive investigation of the synergistic and additive effects of the different growth factors *in vivo* is needed to understand the complex network of hematopoietic regulation and, thus, the potential usefulness of cytokines as new therapeutic agents.

Acknowledgment

The authors acknowledge the rewarding and continued cooperation of Steven Gillis, David L. Urdal, David Cosman, and Christopher C. Henney (Immunex Corporation, Seattle, WA). The authors also thank Karin Markolf, Friedrich Lolkes, Heinrich Kraft, and Astrid Ernst for their expert help.

References

1. Clark, S. C., and Kamen, R. The human hematopoietic colony-stimulating factors. *Science* 236:1229-1237, 1987.
2. Yang, Y. C., Ciarletta, A. B., Temple, P. A., *et al.* Human IL-3 (multi-CSF): Identification by expression cloning of a novel hematopoietic growth factor related to murine IL-3. *Cell* 47:3-10, 1986.

3. Wong, G. G., Temple, P. A., Leary, A. C., *et al.* Human CSF-1: Molecular cloning and expression of 4-kb cDNA encoding the human urinary protein. *Science* 235:1504-1509, 1987.

4. Cantrell, M. A., Anderson, D., Cerretti, D. P., *et al.* Cloning, sequence and expression of a human granulocyte-macrophage colony-stimulating factor. *Proc Natl Acad Sci USA* 82:6250-6254, 1985.

5. Nagata, S., Tsuchiya, M., Asano, S., *et al.* The chromosomal gene structure and two mRNAs for human granulocyte colony-stimulating factor. *EMBO J* 5:575-581, 1986.

6. Antin, J. H., Smith, B. R., Holmes, W., *et al.* Phase I/II study of recombinant human granulocyte-macrophage colony-stimulating factors in aplastic anemia and myelodysplastic syndrome. *Blood* 72:705-713, 1988.

7. Antman, K. S., Griffin, J. D., Elias, A., *et al.* Effect of recombinant human granulocyte-macrophage colony-stimulating factor on chemotherapy-induced myelosuppression. *N Engl J Med* 319:593-598, 1988.

8. Nemunaitis, J., Singer, J. W., Buckner, C. D., *et al.* Use of recombinant human granulocyte-macrophage colony-stimulating factor in autologous marrow transplantation for lymphoid malignancies. *Blood* 72:834-836, 1988.

9. Paquette, R. L., Zhou, J. Y., Yang, Y. C., *et al.* Recombinant gibbon interleukin-3 acts synergistically with recombinant human G-CSF and GM-CSF *in vitro*. *Blood* 71:1596-1600, 1988.

10. Ikebuchi, K., Clark, S. C., Ihle, J. N., *et al.* Granulocyte colony-stimulating factor enhances interleukin-3-dependent proliferation of multipotential hemopoietic progenitors. *Proc Natl Acad Sci USA* 85:3445-3449, 1988.

11. Krumwieh, D., Weinmann, E., and Siebold, B., *et al.* Preclinical studies on synergistic effects of IL-1, IL-3, G-CSF, and GM-CSF in cynomolgus monkeys. In: *Proceedings of the International Conference on Blood Cell Growth Factors: Their Biology and Clinical Application.* 8-12 October 1989, Capri, Italy, in press.

12. Donahue, R. E., Seehra, J., Metzger, M., *et al.* Human IL-3 and GM-CSF act synergistically in stimulating hematopoiesis in primates. *Science* 241:1820-1823, 1988.

13. Valent, P., Geissler, K., Mayer, P., *et al.* The *in vivo* effects of IL-3 and GM-CSF in primates. *Molecular Biotherapy* 1(Suppl):67 (Abstract), 1989.

14. Nicola, N. Why do hematopoietic growth factor receptors interact with each other? *Immunol Today* 8:134-139, 1987.

15. Lopez, A. F., Dyson, P. G., To, B. L., *et al.* Recombinant human interleukin-3 stimulation of hematopoiesis in humans: Loss of responsiveness with differentiation in the neutrophilic myeloid series. *Blood* 72:1797-1804, 1988.

Hematopoietic Injury Complications

Roundtable Discussion
(Questions and discussions were summarized by the book editors.)

Question:

What are the recommendations for using blood products in patients when the need for bone marrow transplantation is not immediately obvious? Are there any recommendations about transfusing those patients initially with related-donor products?

Discussion:

The recommendation is to use random-donor products initially, simply for logistical reasons—they are available at every blood bank throughout the country. There is no evidence that the onset of allosensitization is delayed if blood products donated by family members are used. Anyone who has not had a transfusion should respond equally well to blood products donated by random donors and family members.

All blood products should be irradiated *in vitro* to prevent the occurrence of graft-versus-host disease, which is mediated by transfused mononuclear cells.

Question:

Was the use of packed red blood cells considered for treatment of patients with moderate to severe hematopoietic injury?

Discussion:

Packed red blood cells are recommended when standard clinical criteria suggest the need for transfusion. Packed red cells should be passed through a filter to remove the mononuclear cells that could potentially transmit disease, and should also be irradiated to eliminate immunocompetent leukocytes.

Question:

We discussed treatment strategies for four categories of patients, identified as receiving mild, moderate, severe, and lethal doses of radiation, without giving any specifics as to how casualties can be classified into these groups using objective criteria. There are discrepancies between physical and biological dosimetry, and free-in-air dose measurements are of little, if any, use. How, then, can these categories be defined scientifically?

Discussion:

Given the disagreement in assessing exact dosimetry standards, it may be impossible to state precisely what constitutes mild, moderate, severe, and lethal injury. Rely on biologic dosimetry and arrange for phenotyping when possible. Individuals receiving less than 2 Gy (2 sieverts) would be in the mild group; those receiving 2-5, 6, or 8 Gy, in the moderate group; and those receiving higher doses, in the severe group.

Question:

We assumed that the $LD_{50/60}$ for man without therapy of any kind is about 4.5 Gy of low-LET (linear energy transfer) radiation, measured free in air. What would the $LD_{50/60}$ be with supportive therapy of antibiotics, fluids and electrolyte balancing, platelets, and others?

Discussion:

With timely provision of supportive care that includes reverse isolation (ideally, laminar airflow environment) and administration of antibiotics, fluids, and platelets, the LD_{50} might be raised to approximately 6-7 Gy.

Question:

If hematopoietic growth factors were available, what would be the potential effect of their addition to the support protocol? How high would the $LD_{50/60}$ value be raised?

Discussion:

There is, of course, no clinical experience to use in answering this question. Data from canine studies suggest that the LD_{50} might be somewhat higher, possibly 1-1.5 Gy higher. The application of clinical support (fluids, as required; antibiotics; and fresh, irradiated random donor platelets) can increase the survival of lethally irradiated canines (2.6-3.4 Gy midline tissue dose). The dose reduction factor (DRF) of 1.3 obtained in canines with clinical support corresponds to a human $LD_{50/60}$ dose of 5.85 Gy. Current data using recombinant human granulocyte-macrophage colony-stimulating factor (rhGM-CSF) or recombinant human granulocyte colony-stimulating factor (rhG-CSF) with clinical support suggest that the canine $LD_{50/30}$ can be raised to approximately 4.5 Gy midline tissue dose. This DRF of 1.8 corresponds to an increase to 8.1 Gy for a human $LD_{50/60}$ free-in-air dose.

Question:

Can growth factors be used to treat thrombocytopenia?

Discussion:

The known growth factors, GM-CSF and G-CSF, do not affect platelets. Interleukin-3 is the only factor currently in clinical trials that shows promise in stimulating thrombopoiesis. However, the effect of such a growth factor is likely to take 1-2 weeks to produce the optimum response in platelets. Consequently, it is unlikely that any amount of a hematopoietic growth factor would abrogate the need for platelet transfusions early in the course of hematopoietic injury.

Question:

Presently, what indicators can we use to distinguish between patients who have reversible versus irreversible bone marrow damage?

Discussion:

Hematological parameters in concert with knowledge of the prodromal symptoms should be used to determine the degree of bone marrow damage. The presence of the prodromal symptoms are an indication of the acute radiation syndrome. The onset, severity, and duration of symptoms can be used initially to classify the patients in the radiation categories. If there is no nausea or vomiting, there is little possibility of acute radiation exposure. If there is persistent nausea, vomiting, and diarrhea through 48 hours, the probability of survival after any treatment, other than bone marrow transplantation, is rather remote. In the hematology profile of less severe cases, a moderate depression of lymphocytes may be seen. About 28-30 days after exposure, the nadir of granulocytes and platelets will appear, followed by a leisurely marrow recovery. Between these two categories there will be individuals who have nausea, vomiting, or diarrhea that spontaneously subsides in approximately 24 hours. A good example of this behavior was the course of Japanese soldiers who had rather severe symptomatology on the first day, went back to duty, worked for 3-4 weeks, and then began dying of infection (in the third to fourth week after exposure) and from hemorrhage (in the fifth to seventh week after exposure).

If an individual receives 5 Gy of radiation, and the proposed bone marrow donor is genetically an identical twin, the inclination might be to do the transplant at 5 Gy, especially if the patient is less than 20 years old. If the individual in question is 63 years old, and the proposed donor a completely mismatched uncle, an exposure dose of 8 Gy may be required. In the context of a nuclear war, it is likely that the siblings of the people who are rescuable would likewise be irradiated; that is, a population of persons would likely be living in close proximity to their irradiated relatives. Whereas, in an industrial accident, as in Chernobyl, the residents of Pripyat were plant workers, and their potential donors were likely not irradiated because they lived outside the area of the accident.

Question:

What are the main problems with bone marrow grafting?

Discussion:

Data from the 1940's to the present have shown the discrepancy between physical and biologic dosimetry. In deciding on bone marrow transplantation during the early postexposure period, this uncertainty poses a great problem. If there is any risk in bone marrow transplantation, it is greatest for those receiving a lower dose of radiation.

Extrapolations from radiation exposures in a clinical setting to an accident scenario may be dangerous. For example, a "window of benefit" for bone marrow transplantation for an 8-16 Gy dose may be too large. Receiving 16 Gy in one dose is not the same as receiving it over 4 days, as occurs in radiotherapy. Apart from damage to the bone marrow and the gastrointestinal tract, if such a high dose is not fractionated, there will be serious damage to the lungs, liver, and kidneys. It will be difficult within the first 48-72 hours to assess the damage to these organs.

The grafts may not be accepted, particularly if the marrow is manipulated to remove T cells. For a patient who had low-level radiation exposure (up to 3 Gy), the worst that can happen following an apparently unnecessary bone marrow transplantation is graft rejection, and then the patient's own marrow might recover. Mouse experiments indicating a midlethal dose effect are probably not valid in humans. With a higher radiation dose (for example, 6 Gy), the host may accept the transplant temporarily (for 6-8 weeks), thus providing the host with granulocytes. The host's own marrow may recover by this time, and the host may then reject the transplanted graft.

Animal experiments use both fractionated exposures and single-dose exposure. Single-dose exposure may be compared to a radiation accident where the exposure is somewhat chaotic. In the fractionated exposure, when 1.25 Gy were administered three times a day for 4 days, neutrophils dropped to neutropenic levels by the fourth or fifth day. This finding can be extrapolated to an accident scenario, where marked neutropenia in this time frame would indicate a severe exposure.

It is difficult to conceive of the use of bone marrow transplantation in the aftermath of strategic nuclear weapon detonations. Apart from the logistical problems, the window of benefit is narrow (8-12 Gy); the uncertainty of dose, dose rate, and energy is great, and the clinical symptoms are likely to be highly variable. The experience at Chernobyl indicates that bone marrow transplantation is a more viable option than fetal liver transplantation.

Question:

What is the role of imaging techniques in identifying surviving pockets of bone marrow in nonuniform radiation exposures?

Discussion:

Technicium-labelled iron, which identifies active bone marrow sites, has been used in animal studies and in clinical trials. The value of this technique in a radiation accident is not known. Such imaging may be done better with magnetic resonance. Another technique, radiolabelled antimyeloid antibody, which is used for total-body scanning to determine bone marrow reserves, has not been used.

Question:

Is there an ethical question concerning the risk to bone marrow donors who receive general anesthesia?

Discussion:

Donors do not succumb to anesthetic procedure or other complications. The risk is considered justifiable, especially when the donor is a sibling or a family member.

Question:

What is the status of the national bone marrow registry? What is its interaction with the international bone marrow registry?

Discussion:

There are about 30,000 donors currently registered in the national bone marrow registry. Additionally, there are ties with registries in Great Britain, France, Netherlands, Germany, Austria, Switzerland, and Italy. In a given situation, provided there is enough time, there is about a 35-percent chance of finding an appropriate, identical unrelated donor. Unfortunately, in the case of radiation accidents, it would take too long to locate an appropriate donor. Presently, it can be categorically stated that there is little likelihood for a radiation victim to receive a bone marrow transplant from an unrelated donor.

Question:

What are the long-term outcomes for the patients who were heavily contaminated in the Brazilian accident?

Discussion:

This depends on many factors. The "dose commitment" for each patient is determined in such a way that the probability of getting cancer can be roughly estimated for each individual. In general, those who were exposed externally present a greater risk of stochastic effects, compared to those with only internal contamination. This subject is one of the most important challenges to be faced by radiation medicine specialists and epidemiologists.

Question:

What were the signs and symptoms of anoxia in the Brazilian accident patients?

Discussion:

At least three patients showed signs of anoxia during the critical phase of the hematopoietic syndrome. This was determined by peripheral signs (cyanosis of the extremities and mucosa) and tachypnea, which were both observed in all patients. Arterial blood gas measurements were not performed. Anoxia was caused by infectious complications (pneumonitis interfering with oxygen exchange through alveolar membranes) in two patients.

Infectious Complications

Infections in Radiation Accidents

An Overview

Stephen C. Schimpff

Introduction

Although the radiation-injured patient may develop cellular immune deficiency or humoral immune deficiency, the major predisposing factor to infection, especially in the short term, is granulocytopenia. Infections associated with intravascular devices and as a consequence of blood product infusions occur too. As a result, most infections are caused by the aerobic gram-negative rods *Escherichia coli, Pseudomonas aeruginosa,* and *Klebsiella pneumoniae,* along with the gram-positive cocci *Staphylococcus aureus, Staphylococcus epidermidis,* and *Streptococcus* species. The sites of infection are principally the oral cavity and associated structures (for example, sinusitis, periodontitis, pharyngitis, and local mucositis); the distal third of the esophagus; the lungs (pneumonitis); the colon (bacteremia related to translocation); perianal lesions; and sites of skin damage, such as vascular catheter exit sites. Other infections, especially bacteremias, are associated with the catheter itself. Most infections are caused by organisms colonizing the patient, and more than half of these are acquired during hospitalization. Treatment of infections during granulocytopenia has been discussed in detail.[1,2]

It is essential from the diagnostic, therapeutic, and preventive perspectives to separate the granulocytopenic patient population into two groups: those with moderate degrees of granulocytopenia and those with essentially no circulating granulocytes ($< 100/\mu$L) for prolonged periods. In patients in the latter group, the normal signs of inflammation are so muted that fever may be the only early indication of serious infection. These patients are at greater risk of bacteremia, especially gram-negative rod bacteremia, and mortality is high even when empiric antimicrobials are administered promptly. These same patients may or may not benefit from a combination of active agents rather

S. C. SCHIMPFF, American Cancer Society Professor of Oncology, University of Maryland Cancer Center, Executive Vice President, University of Maryland Medical System, Baltimore, Maryland 21201.

Treatment of Radiation Injuries, Edited by
D. Browne *et al.,* Plenum Press, New York, 1990

than from monotherapy. Finally, the patient with profound, persistent granulocytopenia requires aggressive approaches to prevent infection. Among these approaches are attempts to improve host defenses; close attention to detail in the use of invasive procedures, especially intravascular catheters; attempts to reduce the acquisition of new organisms, especially by careful handwashing and the use of a low-microbial-content diet; and attempts to suppress colonizing potential pathogens, preferably by a selective approach so as to preserve alimentary canal anaerobic flora.

Factors Increasing the Probability of Infection

Iatrogenic factors, cellular immune deficiency, humoral immune deficiency, and especially granulocytopenia, in concert with shifts of microbial flora and damage to normal anatomic barriers to organism penetration, predispose the patient to infection following irradiation. In addition, trauma has multiple adverse consequences to the normal host defense mechanisms against infection.

Iatrogenic Factors

The major iatrogenic factors are intravascular catheters, urinary catheters, contamination from administration of blood products, and the adverse effects of trauma and drugs. They are all well-known problems, but a brief comment regarding Hickman and similar venous access devices is pertinent.

The commonly used right atrial catheters are made of barium-impregnated silicone rubber, are about 90 cm long, and have a dacron felt cuff 30 cm from the external end. When inserted subcutaneously, this cuff is positioned about 2 cm above the skin exit site. During a 10-year period at the University of Maryland Cancer Center, exit site infections were found in 160 of 593 patients who had 690 catheters placed. Exit site infections developed at any time from day 1 to day 1,210; the median time to onset was 80 days. Although 100 of these patients were granulocytopenic, 60 patients had more than 1,000 granulocytes/μL at the onset of their exit site infections. Documentation of the etiologic organism was possible in only 59 instances. *Staphylococcus aureus* was the most common pathogen, distantly followed by *Pseudomonas aeruginosa* and *Staphylococcus epidermidis* (table 1). Over time, it became apparent that catheters did not need to be removed when exit site infections developed. Systemic antimicrobial therapy directed at the etiologic organism, when it was known, proved to be successful in most patients, including 12 who had bacteremia.

Tunnel infections proved to be substantially different from exit site infections and, with only a few exceptions, did not appear to originate as exit site infections. Tunnel infections occurred in 46 of the 690 catheter placements (median 70 days) after placement (range 2 to 727 days), and were more common in double

Table 1. Factors Increasing the Probability of Infection and Types of Organisms Causing Infection

Factor	Type of organism
Intravascular access catheters	*Staphylococcus aureus* *Staphylococcus epidermidis*
Cellular immune deficiency	Bacteria: *Listeria monocytogenes* *Legionella pneumophila* *Mycobacteria* *Nocardia asteroides* Viruses: Herpes simplex Varicella-zoster Cytomegalovirus Epstein-Barr virus Fungi: *Histoplasma capsulatum* *Coccidioides immitis* *Cryptococcus neoformans* *Candida* species Protozoa: *Pneumocystis carinii* *Toxoplasma gondii* Helminth: *Strongyloides stercoralis*
Humoral immune deficiency	*Streptococcus pneumoniae* *Hemophilus influenzae* *Neisseria meningitidis*
Granulocytopenia	Aerobic gram-positive cocci: *Staphylococcus aureus* *Staphylococcus epidermidis* *Streptococcus* species Aerobic gram-negative bacilli: *Escherichia coli* *Pseudomonas aeruginosa* *Klebsiella pneumoniae* Yeasts: *Candida albicans* *Candida tropicalis* Fungi: *Aspergillus flavus* *Aspergillus fumigatus*

lumen catheters (median 30 days) than in single lumen catheters (median 98 days). Most infections (32 of 46) occurred when the patient was granulocytopenic. Microbiological documentation, which was possible in 20 of the 46 tunnel infections, showed that *Staphylococcus aureus* was the most common isolated pathogen and the most common cause of tunnel-associated bacteremia. During the 10-year study period, 397 bacteremias occurred among the 690 catheter placements. Obviously, in a population largely dominated by patients with acute leukemia, most bacteremias were not catheter related but arose from the common sites of infections in these patients, such as pneumonias and perirectal and perianal lesions. However, 13 bacteremias were associated with exit site infections, and 12 were associated with tunnel infections. It is unclear how many of the remaining 372 bacteremias were Hickman catheter associated. In many cases, when *Staphylococcus epidermidis* was the bacteremic organism, it was assumed to be related to the catheter, but in only 8 of 62 instances did we find it necessary to remove the catheter. We based our decision on persistence of bacteremia in the face of appropriate therapy (vancomycin). Only rarely were *Staphylococcus aureus, Pseudomonas aeruginosa*, or enteric gram-negative bacilli thought to be catheter related, and in only 7 of 168 such bacteremias were the catheters removed on the assumption that the infection could not be controlled otherwise.

Cellular Immune Deficiency

Cellular immune deficiency leads to infection with an array of organisms, many of which are obligate intracellular parasites (table 1). They include the bacteria *Listeria monocytogenes, Legionella pneumophila, Mycobacteria*, and *Nocardia asteroides*; the viruses herpes simplex, varicella-zoster, cytomegalovirus, and Epstein-Barr virus; the fungi *Histoplasma capsulatum, Coccidioides immitis, Cryptococcus neoformans*, and *Candida* species; the protozoa *Pneumocystis carinii, Toxoplasma gondii*, and others; and the helminth *Strongyloides stercoralis*. These organisms tend to cause infection frequently in patients with severe cellular immune deficiency (such as those with acquired immune deficiency syndrome). Infection is less frequent in patients who have lesser degrees of cellular immune deficiency (such as those with Hodgkin's disease or renal transplantation) and only intermediately frequent in patients with bone marrow transplantation.

Humoral Immune Deficiency

Some months after bone marrow transplantation, humoral immune deficiency is found in patients with multiple myeloma and chronic lymphocytic leukemia. The deficiency leads to infections with the encapsulated pyogenic organisms, most notably with *Streptococcus pneumoniae*, but occasionally with *Hemophilus influenzae* and *Neisseria meningitidis*. Children who have a splenectomy before age 10 are at particularly high risk for the overwhelming pneumococcal sepsis syndrome. This syndrome is also seen in adults at any time after a splenectomy, although much less frequently.

Granulocytopenia

The major short- and long-term predisposing factor to consider in association with radiation injuries is granulocytopenia, which alone is usually not sufficient to lead to infection; rather, infection tends to occur at sites of the body where there has been some breach of a normal anatomic barrier that otherwise prevents microbial invasion. Further, in any ill individual, shifts of microbial flora cause changes in mucosal and skin surfaces. Of particular importance is the change of oral flora, which will tend toward aerobic gram-negative bacilli in any ill patient, even in the absence of antimicrobial therapy. This tendency has significant implications for the types of infections that occur in the mouth, oral pharynx, respiratory tract, and esophagus. These changes in oral flora apparently have to do with changes in the mucosal binding (perhaps related to fibronectin) in the epithelial cells. Skin flora may also change, and aerobic gram-negative bacilli may become frequent, if not predominant, in the axillae and inguinal regions. Once antibiotic therapy has been administered, the flora of the oral cavity, the lower alimentary canal, and the skin will change further because of colonization by resistant strains of bacteria and yeasts.

The organisms that most commonly cause infection in the granulocytopenic patient are the aerobic gram-positive cocci *Staphylococcus aureus*, *Staphylococcus epidermidis*, and *Streptococcus* species, and the aerobic gram-negative rods *Escherichia coli*, *Pseudomonas aeruginosa*, and *Klebsiella pneumoniae*. Although other aerobic bacteria can and do cause infection, they are distinctly in the minority, compared with these six organisms, which represent more than 80 percent of bacterial infections. In these patients, who tend to be hospitalized for prolonged periods, acquired organisms cause 50 percent or more of infections, and acquired gram-negative rods are more likely to be resistant to commonly used antimicrobials. Among patients who have received antibiotics, infections with yeasts and fungi—particularly *Candida albicans*, *Candida tropicalis*, *Aspergillus flavus*, and *Aspergillus fumigatus*—become more frequent.

The incidence of infection is inversely related to the absolute granulocyte count. As shown in figure 1, most severe infections and nearly all bacteremias occur when the patient has < 100 granulocytes/μL. Bacteremias are most prevalent in patients with prolonged periods of bone marrow aplasia. These periods are critical points in the consideration of diagnosis, prevention, and therapy of infections during granulocytopenia. First, diagnosis: the patient with aplastic marrow and no circulating granulocytes has such impaired inflammatory response that the usual signs of inflammation (heat, redness, swelling, and pain) are muted at best. Nevertheless, the site of infection can usually be defined

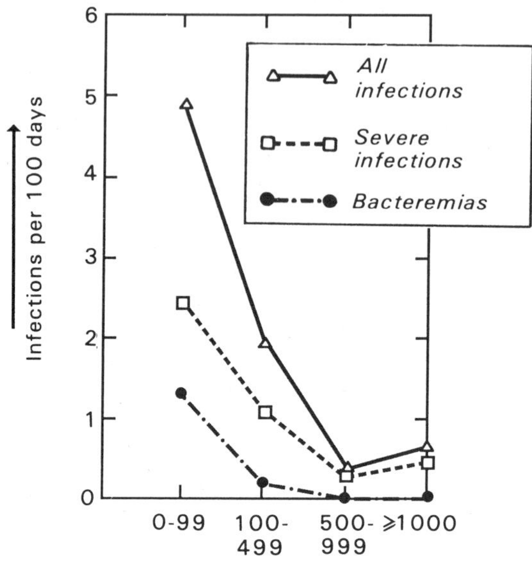

Figure 1. Incidence of infection in patients with acute nonlymphocytic leukemia during induction therapy.

by means of careful, repeated examinations and close attention to patient history, along with repeated chest x rays. Second, prevention: the only patients at high risk of severe infection and bacteremia are those with essentially no circulating granulocytes; they are also the only patients for whom intensive approaches at prophylaxis, such as the use of oral nonabsorbable antibiotics or selective microbial decontamination, would be appropriate. Third, therapy: it is essential in reviewing approaches to infection therapy to consider individuals with no circulating granulocytes separately from those with modest degrees of granulocytopenia because the prognostic implications for the two groups are dramatically different.

Bone Marrow Transplantation

The patient with bone marrow transplantation is a good model for the other types of predisposing factors. Immediately after conditioning for the marrow transplant, the patient is profoundly granulocytopenic for 14-20 days or more. During this period, infections common to aplasia will predominate—namely, gram-negative and gram-positive aerobic bacterial infections and occasionally yeast and fungal infections caused by *Candida* and *Aspergillus*. Herpes simplex infections also occur during this period, but within a few weeks other infections commonly associated with cellular immune deficiency begin to take precedence as the granulocyte count recovers. During this period, the same time in which acute graft-versus-host disease and its attendant therapy occur, infections are caused by cytomegalovirus, adenovirus, and *Pneumocystis carinii*. Later, when the patient may have chronic graft-versus-host disease, varicella-zoster frequently causes infection, and infection with *Streptococcus pneumoniae* and possibly *Hemophilus influenzae* may occur in association with diminished opsonizing antibodies. Because these patients frequently have Hickman or similar intravascular access devices in place, especially during the first few months after the transplant, catheter-related infections are commonplace. Especially common catheter-related infections are caused by *Staphylococcus epidermidis* at the exit site, along the tunnel, or as a result of internal catheter colonization with a biofilm. Because patients with chronic graft-versus-host disease tend to receive multiple blood product transfusions, they may become infected with one of the hepatitis viruses (most commonly non-A non-B hepatitis), and occasionally they may become infected with cytomegalovirus related to blood product transfusions. In addition, because these patients receive multiple courses of antibiotics, it is common to find *Clostridium difficile* colonization of the colon with associated diarrhea or even severe enterocolitis.

Infection Therapy During Granulocytopenia

Among patients with granulocytopenia who develop fever, approximately 20 percent have a bacteremia, another 20 percent have a microbiologically documented infection without an associated bacteremia, 20 percent have a clinically documented infection (i.e., the site of infection is documented but the pathogen is not), about 20 percent fall into the category of fever of unknown origin, and a final 20 percent have a fever of noninfectious origin.

Among profoundly granulocytopenic patients, the onset of gram-negative bacteremia is an adverse prognostic sign unless the patient is treated promptly with appropriate antimicrobials. Indeed, about 50 percent of patients die within the first 24-48 hours if they have been treated with inappropriate antibiotics or simply not treated. There are at least three issues to consider in making a decision about appropriate empiric therapy (table 2). First, one needs to be aware of the recent patterns of infection (i.e., types of organisms and sites of infection) in the individual. Second, one needs to know the current treatment facility susceptibility patterns (i.e., types of antibiotics appropriate for the specific types of bacteria with consideration of resistant bacteria in that facility). Third, it is important to know the current susceptibility patterns of infection in the specific unit where the patient is being treated. Because more than 50 percent of infections are caused by acquired organisms, it follows that knowledge of recent susceptibility patterns is helpful in selecting an appropriate antimicrobial regimen. If the patient remains febrile after therapy has been instituted, there are a number of issues to consider in altering therapy.

Results from published literature on empiric antibiotic therapy show that 20 percent of patients will have a bacteremia, half of which will be caused by gram-negative bacilli. On the one hand, this 10 percent is a substantial

Table 2. Empiric Issues to Consider
in Infection Therapy

Initial choice of therapy:

- Recent patterns of infection in the individual
- Current treatment facility susceptibility patterns
- Current susceptibility patterns of infections in the specific unit where the patient is being treated

Modifying therapy for the patient with continued fever:

- Results of daily history and examination
- Previous recent antibiotic therapy
- Duration of granulocytopenia to date and likelihood of future duration
- Presence of vascular access device
- Use of bone marrow transplant
- Previous infections, especially viral or protozoan
- Results of surveillance cultures
- Recognition of recent treatment facility patterns

number at high risk of mortality if not treated appropriately and quickly. On the other hand, 10 percent is a relatively small percentage of patients at high risk of mortality when data are compared among regimens. For example, in the most recent trial by the European Organization for Research on the Treatment of Cancer, International Antimicrobial Therapy (EORTC IV), 1,074 febrile episodes associated with granulocytopenia were studied. However, as one would expect, only 90 patients had a gram-positive bacteremia, and 129 had a gram-negative bacteremia.

Approximately 30 entries of gram-positive bacteremia and 40 of gram-negative bacteremia were made in each of the three regimens under study. Given that the bacteremias were caused by a variety of gram-positive or gram-negative bacteria and arose from a variety of sites, (for example, pneumonia and perianal fissures), comparisons were difficult, although the study population was exceptionally large. Furthermore, there is a marked difference in prognosis between patients who have profound, persistent granulocytopenia and those whose bone marrow is regenerating, causing the granulocyte count to recover. For example, at our institution, among 75 consecutive patients with gram-negative bacteremias that occurred when the granulocyte count was less than $100/\mu L$, those who had a recovering granulocyte count had an excellent response to a two-drug empiric regimen; 29 of 34 patients (85 percent) responded. However, in those patients with profound, persistent granulocytopenia, only 12 of 41 patients (29 percent) responded to the two-drug regimen.

The key point is that in the absence of any circulating granulocytes, even promptly administered and effective antibiotics have a relatively low rate of infection resolution. On the other hand, with the return of granulocytes, the response rate for patients with gram-negative bacteremia is excellent, as has been borne out in a number of large-scale investigations. As another example, the EORTC III trial found that 28 of 46 patients (61 percent) recovered with prompt empiric antibiotic therapy in the setting of gram-negative bacteremia and recovery of circulating granulocytes. However, only 9 of 34 infections (26 percent) were resolved when the granulocyte count remained at $< 100/\mu L$.

Preventing Infection During Granulocytopenia

Infections in granulocytopenic patients can be reduced by attention to four key issues: improving host defenses, reducing invasive procedures, suppressing potential pathogens, and reducing organism acquisition.

Improving Host Defenses

There are relatively few pertinent vaccines for patients in this setting, although the influenza vaccine will prevent serious bacterial superinfections as well as influenza. Research does not suggest that direct intravenous infusion of gamma globulin will substantively reduce the incidence or severity of infection. Granulocyte transfusions have been effective in reducing serious infections, especially gram-negative rod bacteremia, but the technical requirements and the adverse effects are sufficient to make this approach generally impractical. Perhaps most important during the past decade has been the reduction in the amount of time required for the patient with acute leukemia to achieve complete remission following combination chemotherapy; the number of days of granulocytopenia and, therefore, the risk of infection have been markedly reduced. A few years ago, lithium was suggested as an approach to improve the number of circulating granulocytes. It proved to be only marginally useful at best, however, because its effect is only to augment release of leukocytes from the bone marrow, not to encourage more rapid bone marrow production. Colony-stimulating factors (CSF's) that are currently under investigation, such as granulocyte CSF and granulocyte-macrophage CSF, have potential for stimulating bone marrow activity and reducing the duration and/or intensity of granulocytopenia. Unlike granulocyte transfusions and lithium, they may prove to have a substantial role in improving host defenses and, therefore, in preventing infection.

Reducing Invasive Procedures

Particularly important is meticulous attention to the use of Hickman and related vascular access catheters. Careful attention to dental hygiene is important to reduce oral complications of granulocytopenia and concomitant radiation or chemotherapy, particularly to prevent exacerbations of chronic periodontitis.

Suppressing Potential Pathogens

The acquisition of potential pathogens can be reduced, but previous standard methods of reverse isolation are of little value. Gowns, masks, and booties probably have little relevance, because most organisms are acquired from the air, water, food, and (primarily) contact with the hands of personnel. Routine reverse isolation does not deal with air, water, or food problems. The simple procedure is to provide an appropriate water supply and a low-microbial-content diet. Many common foodstuffs, such as green leafy vegetables, are normally colonized with the organisms most likely to cause infection in this patient population, namely, *Pseudomonas aeruginosa*, *Klebsiella pneumoniae*, and *Escherichia coli*. Many citrus fruits are colonized with *Candida* and *Torulopsis*, and tomatoes are almost universally colonized internally with *Pseudomonas aeruginosa*. The contact issue can be dealt with by using gloves, but simple handwashing, perhaps with an antiseptic such as chlorhexidine, is adequate. The air is more problematic. Laminar airflow rooms that use high-efficiency particle air filtration will essentially eliminate microbes in the ambient air; the technology is expensive, however, and it requires the patient to be confined to a limited area. Simpler air filtration devices can be placed in individual patient rooms and can clean the air substantially, although not completely.

Reducing Acquisition of Organisms

Reducing the acquisition of organisms from the hospital may benefit high-risk patients by suppressing their colonizing flora. One approach is to use oral nonabsorbable antibiotics (such as gentamicin, vancomycin, and nystatin) designed to suppress the gram-negative rods, the gram-positive cocci, and the yeasts colonizing the alimentary canal. When such an approach is used, a liquid preparation is necessary to suppress the oral organisms. The oral flora will have shifted toward gram-negative bacilli, and these organisms cause infection not only in the oral cavity but in the esophagus and respiratory tract as well. The use of oral nonabsorbable antibiotics reduces infections that arise from organisms colonizing along the alimentary canal. However, the patient at high risk of developing infection is the one with $< 100\ \mu L$ circulating granulocytes for some prolonged period of time. It makes no sense to give this type of regimen to a patient with modest levels of granulocytopenia or even to a patient with profound granulocytopenia of short duration. Further, these regimens take 7-10 days to achieve an adequate effect. Therefore, they need to be started before preparation for bone marrow transplantation or before the granulocyte count falls to dangerous levels. Even when these caveats are followed, there can be problems with development of resistance and with tolerance because of the unpleasant taste. If a patient discontinues the regimen during the course of prophylaxis, a major adverse effect may result because the aerobic gram-negative rods regrow rapidly along the colon with subsequent invasion and bacteremia.

Another approach to microbial suppression is to repress only the aerobic gram-positive and gram-negative rods and yeasts while attempting to preserve the anaerobic flora (which assist the body in resisting colonization by newly acquired organisms). Trimethoprim/sulfamethoxazole (TMP/SMX) was perhaps the first regimen to be used in this fashion, and it gained wide acceptance. TMP/SMX has the disadvantage of having no effect against *Pseudomonas aeruginosa*, and some investigations have suggested that it may prolong the period of granulocytopenia. With the advent of the new quinolones active against *Pseudomonas aeruginosa*, interest has shifted toward norfloxacin, ciprofloxacin, and related compounds. These drugs affect only the aerobic flora and leave the anaerobic organisms intact. Early reports suggest a high degree of efficacy. To be effective, however, any regimen must be followed regularly. Pizzo et al.[3] noted that when compliance was essentially total, the frequency of fever or infection was substantially reduced. Among placebo patients, 32 percent who took the placebo exactly as prescribed developed fever or infection, whereas 44 percent of those who complied only partially and 100 percent of those whose compliance was poor developed fever or infection. These figures suggest that many factors related to reducing infection are not well understood, but seem to relate to the compliance of the patient. They also suggest that it is worthwhile for the medical and nursing staff to spend time with the patient to explain how to prevent infection and that decreased infection results in decreased morbidity and mortality.

References

1. Therapy for Immunocompromised Patients. Combined Symposium Proceedings, Kyoto, Japan. S. C. Schimpff, J. Klastersky, and H. Gaya, Eds. *Am J Med* 80(5C), 1986.
2. Schimpff, S. C. Infections in the compromised host—an overview. In: *Principles and Practice of Infectious Diseases*. 3rd edition. G. L. Mandell, R. G. Douglas, Jr., and J. E. Bennett, Eds. Churchill Livingstone, New York, 1990, pp. 2258-2265.
3. Pizzo, P. A., and Schimpff, S. C. Strategies for the prevention of infection in the myelosuppressed cancer patient. *Cancer Treat Rep* 67:223-234, 1983.

Antibiotics in Postirradiation Infection

Itzhak Brook

Mechanism of Bacterial Infection

Increasing doses of radiation are associated with progressively higher mortality rates in animals,[1-3] largely because of their increased susceptibility to various endogenous or exogenous pathogens.[3] After irradiation, enteric organisms were recovered from lymphatic organs as well as from the bloodstream of these animals.[4]

Organisms were detected more often in the spleen, liver, or blood of mice exposed to higher doses of cobalt-60 gamma radiation. Bacteria were recovered in 3 of 100 mice at 7 Gy, in 13 of 100 at 8 Gy, in 23 of 90 at 9 Gy, and in 34 of 87 at 10 Gy. A relationship was also found between the dose of radiation and the type of bacteria causing sepsis.[4] *Escherichia coli* (anaerobic cocci and *Bacteroides* species) were more often isolated in animals given 10 Gy, whereas *Staphylococcus aureus* was more often recovered in those given 9 Gy (figure 1). Most bacterial isolates were recovered between days 9 and 13 after irradiation, probably because of the maximal effects of the combination of leukopenia, immunosuppression, and failure of mucosal barriers against bacterial translocation at subsequent infection that occur on these days.[3,5-7]

The biological effects induced by the combination of trauma and irradiation act synergistically and may have significant impact on the host's ability to survive. The response of the irradiated host to wound infection was investigated in an animal model.[8] Mice irradiated with 6.5 Gy showed increased local susceptibility in the wound to challenge with bacteria commonly found in wound and soft tissue infections. These organisms included *S. aureus*, *E. coli*, and *Streptococcus pyogenes*. Quantitative cultures of the infected wounds showed 10^3 to 10^4 more viable organisms in irradiated and wounded mice compared to nonirradiated and wounded mice (figure 2).

I. BROOK, Experimental Hematology Department, Armed Forces Radiobiology Research Institute, Bethesda, Maryland 20814-5145.

Treatment of Radiation Injuries, Edited by
D. Browne *et al.,* Plenum Press, New York, 1990

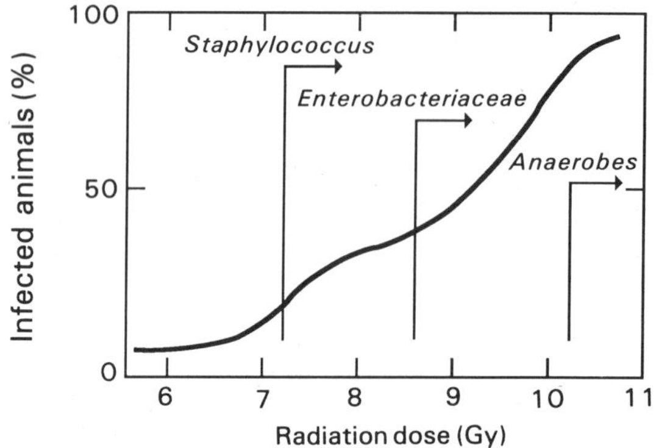

Figure 1. Microorganisms recovered from irradiated mice in relation to radiation dose. (Previously published in *Radiation Research*, Volume 115, July 1988.)

The length of time between the irradiation, wounding, and challenging had a significant effect on the wound infection. Inoculating the organisms into the mice on and after the third day following the irradiation caused the most severe infections. This increased susceptibility coincided with the development of postirradiation leukopenia and thrombocytopenia. Increased susceptibility related to leukopenia was also observed by Schechmeister et al.[9] and Kaplan et al.,[10] who found that animals were more susceptible to generalized infection at 3-7 days after irradiation.

The severity of the susceptibility to local infections was directly correlated with the radiation dose. When mice were infected with a constant number of *S. aureus* after exposure to cobalt-60 radiation and wounding, infection was noticed only when the animals were exposed to a dose of radiation higher than 7 Gy.[8]

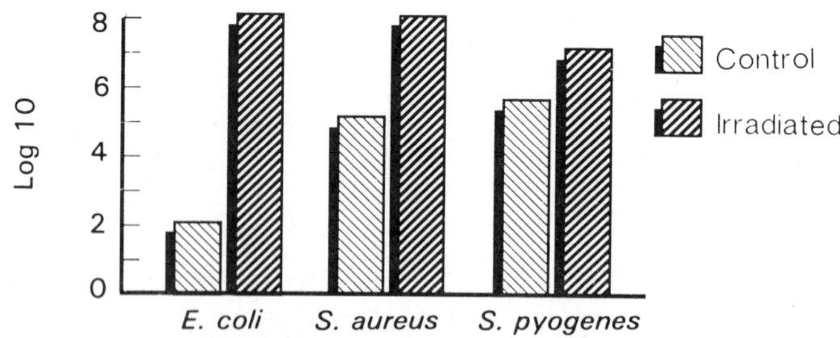

Figure 2. Number of bacteria recovered in infected wounds in control (nonirradiated) and irradiated mice 5 days after irradiation. (Previously published in *Radiation Research*, Volume 115, July 1988.)

Antimicrobial Therapy

The management of infections with antimicrobials in severely immunocompromised subjects is particularly difficult. The efficacy of antimicrobial therapy, mostly with streptomycin, in reducing the mortality of sublethally irradiated animals was demonstrated in the 1950's.[11,12] Although antimicrobial therapy alone controlled the bacteremia, it did not prevent death in lethally irradiated animals.[12,13]

Brook *et al.*[14] administered gentamicin to lethally irradiated mice and were able to reduce the systemic spread of *Enterobacteriaceae* but not of anaerobes. However, even the coadministration of metronidazole (effective only against anaerobic bacteria) did not prevent bacteremia due to anaerobes and mortality. Therapy of wound infection in mice with penicillin and gentamicin prevented bacteremia, but was only partially effective in eliminating local infection with *S. aureus, E. coli,* and *K. pneumoniae.*[8]

Although antimicrobials do not express their maximal effect in the irradiated host, their proper use is essential in controlling local and systemic bacterial infections. The shortcoming of antimicrobial therapy probably results from the impaired immune system, which is needed to eradicate the organisms completely.

No large-scale clinical studies have established the principles of managing patients exposed to radiation. However, experience gained in caring for patients accidentally exposed to radiation indicates that the infections and their management are similar to those for patients who are granulocytopenic because of chemotherapy, immunotherapy, or therapeutic irradiation. Early empirical broad-spectrum antibiotic therapy has become standard practice in the management of these patients, and has contributed to their improved outcomes.[15] As soon as accurate microbiological identification is available, specific antimicrobial therapy is instituted.

Preliminary reports demonstrated that most patients exposed to sublethal alpha, beta, and gamma radiation at the Chernobyl nuclear power plant accident eventually regained normal neutrophils.[16] Until normal neutrophils are regained, it is important to provide patients with adequate antimicrobial therapy against invading endogenous or exogenous bacteria.

A variety of microorganisms from different sources can cause infections in the immunocompromised host. These include organisms of the endogenous flora of the oral cavity, upper respiratory and gastrointestinal (GI) tracts, and skin. Some of the organisms are part of the normal flora before immuno-suppression; others tend to colonize the mucous surfaces after the immune system is depleted. Nosocomial infections can be acquired from the community or the environment as well as from blood products, catheters, and other devices.

Chemoprophylaxis of Enteric Sources of Systemic Infection

Because the GI tract aerobic and facultative bacterial flora are the major sources of infection in immunocompromised patients,[15] a logical approach to reducing the incidence of infection is to suppress only the endogenous GI gram-negative flora,[17-19] while preserving the normal anaerobic gut flora. This approach was illustrated in studies that demonstrated the adverse effects to antimicrobials that suppress the anaerobic flora.[14,20]

After irradiation, the number of aerobic and anaerobic components of the gut flora decrease. This decline is followed by a rapid increase in the number of aerobic and facultative flora (figure 3).[14] Because exposure to high levels of radiation also induces severe changes in the GI mucosa, *Enterobacteriaceae* may easily penetrate the damaged mucosa. Antimicrobials that suppress anaerobes can reduce the number of anaerobes normally observed in all irradiated hosts and may have deleterious effects on the irradiated host. Brook et al.[14] demonstrated that metronidazole facilitates mortality in lethally irradiated mice. Mice treated with metronidazole were all dead by the 9th day after irradiation, whereas untreated irradiated mice were all dead by the 17th day. The recovery of *Enterobacteriaceae* from the tissues of mice treated with metronidazole was associated with a more rapid increase in the number of aerobic and facultative organisms, compared to untreated irradiated mice. This event followed the decline in the number of the GI anaerobic flora induced by metronidazole.

Antimicrobial agents effective against a wide spectrum of microorganisms may, however, be needed to treat severe infections, especially those associated

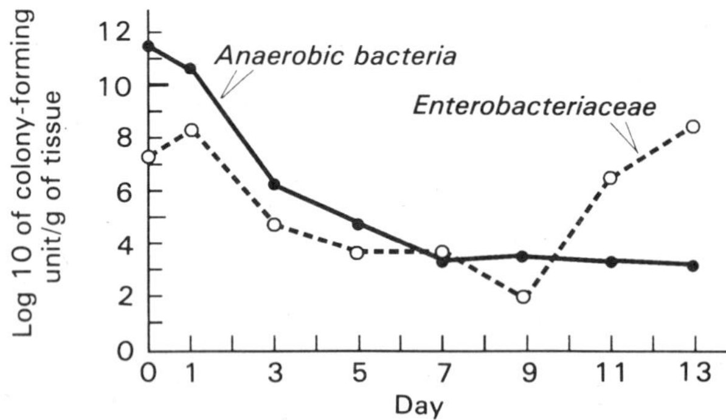

Figure 3. Changes in aerobic and facultative flora in ileum of mice after lethal irradiation (10 Gy). (Previously published in *Radiation Research*, Volume 115, July 1988.)

with intra-abdominal trauma. Further studies are needed to provide guidance in the use of these agents in the irradiated host and to devise therapies that will circumvent or overcome their deleterious effects on the anaerobic GI flora.

Selective decontamination of the GI tract, a technique used to eradicate only the aerobic gram-negative bacilli, has gained increased interest.[21] This approach uses trimethoprim/sulfamethoxazole (TMP/SMX) or quinolones. The systemic absorption of these agents also eradicates gram-negative organisms that might reach the bloodstream.

Several studies have shown conflicting data on the efficacy of TMP/SMX in reducing the infection rate in granulocytopenic patients.[22-25] The newly introduced quinolones have promising potential for use in selective decontamination. These agents exhibit broad antimicrobial activity against aerobic gram-positive and gram-negative bacteria, especially against *Enterobacteriaceae* and *Pseudomonas aeruginosa*,[26] and have limited activity against anaerobic bacteria.

We have found that oral administration of the quinolones pefloxacin, ofloxacin, and ciprofloxacin prolonged the survival of irradiated mice (I. Brook and T. B. Elliott, unpublished data) and was synergistic with glucan, an immunomodulator (M. Patchen, I. Brook, and T. B. Elliott, unpublished data). Further studies are needed to compare the efficacy of quinolones with other modalities in achieving selective decontamination in the immunocompromised host. The quinolones may also be used for therapy of systemic infections caused by aerobic gram-negative or gram-positive bacteria in the immunocompromised host.[27]

Summary

Therapy using antibiotics is only one component of the complex task of managing persons exposed to radiation or persons with combined injury. In these situations, the infecting organisms may be related to the circumstance and the site of the body injured. A synergy between the radiation effects and the physical injury may be more immunosuppressive than single injuries and may induce a higher rate of complications and mortality.[28]

Antimicrobial agents by themselves have a limited role in managing infections in the immunocompromised host, and their success rate in the eradication of infection is much lower than in the immunocompetent host.[15] It is, therefore, imperative that the immune system be protected by the use of radioprotectants and/or stimulated by use of immunomodulators. However, the use of these agents is still experimental, and more research should be done to establish their potential use in irradiated hosts.

References

1. Gordon, L. E., Ruml, D., Hahne, J. H., et al. Studies on susceptibilities to infection following ionizing irradiation. IV. The pathogenesis of the endogenous bacteremia in mice. *J Exp Med* 102:413-424, 1955.
2. Bennett, L. R., Rekers, P. E., and Howland, J. Influence of infection on hematological effects and mortality following mid-lethal roentgen irradiation. *Radiology* 57:99-105, 1951.
3. Benacerraf, B. Influence of irradiation on resistance to infection. *Bacteriol Rev* 24:35-40, 1960.
4. Brook, I., Walker, R. I., and MacVittie, T. J. Effects of radiation dose on the recovery of aerobic and anaerobic bacteria from mice. *Can J Microbiol* 37:719-722, 1966.
5. Carter, P. B., and Collins, F. M. The route of enteric infection in normal mice. *J Exp Med* 139:1189-1203, 1974.
6. Miller, C. P. The effect of irradiation on natural resistance to infection. *Ann NY Acad Sci* 66:250-291, 1956.
7. Collins, F. M. Mucosal defenses against *Salmonella* infection in the mouse. *J Infect Dis* 129:503-519, 1956.
8. Brook, I., and Elliott, T. B. Treatment of wound sepsis in irradiated mice. *Int J Radiat Biol* 56:75-82, 1989.
9. Schechmeister, I. L., Bond, V. P., and Swift, M. N. The susceptibility of irradiated mice to infection as a function of post-irradiation time. *J Immunol* 68:87-95, 1952.
10. Kaplan, H. W., Speck, R. S., and Jawetz, F. Impairment of antimicrobial defenses following total body irradiation of mice. *J Lab Clin Med* 40:682-691, 1952.
11. Hammond, C. W. The treatment of postirradiation infection. *Radiat Res* 1:448-458, 1954.
12. Hammond, C. W., Vogel, H. H., Clark, H. W., et al. The effect of streptomycin therapy in mice irradiated with fast neutrons. *Radiat Res* 2:359-360, 1953.
13. Miller, C. P., Hammond, C. W., Tompkins, M., et al. Treatment of postirradiation infection with antibiotics; an experimental study on mice. *J Lab Clin Med* 39:462-479, 1952.
14. Brook, I., Walker, R. I., and MacVittie, T. J. Effect of antimicrobial therapy on the gut flora and bacterial infection in irradiated mice. *Int J Radiat Biol* 5:709-716, 1988.
15. Bodey, G. P. Infection in cancer patients: A continuing association. *Am J Med* 81(Suppl 1A):11-26, 1986.
16. Gale, R. P. Immediate medical consequences of nuclear accidents: Lessons from Chernobyl. *JAMA* 285:625-628, 1987.
17. EORTC Gnotobiotic Group. Protective isolation and antimicrobial decontamination in patients with high susceptibility to infection. *Infection* 6:175-191, 1978.
18. Reiter, B., Gee, T., Young, L., et al. Use of oral antibiotics during remission induction in adult patients with acute nonlymphoblastic leukemias (ANLL). *Clin Res* 21:652, 1973.
19. Storring, R. A., Jameson, B., McElwain, T. J., et al. Oral nonabsorbed antibiotics prevent infection in acute nonlymphoblastic leukemia. *Lancet* II:837-840, 1977.
20. Berg, R. D. Promotion of the translocation of enteric bacteria from the gastrointestinal tracts of mice by oral treatment with penicillin, clindamycin, or metronidazole. *Infect Immun* 33:854-861, 1981.
21. van der Waaij, O., Hofstra, H., and Wiegersma, N. Effect of beta-lactam antibiotics on the resistance of the digestive tract of mice to colonization. *J Infect Dis* 146:417-422, 1982.
22. Bender, J. F., Schimpff, S. C., Young, V. M., et al. A comparative trial of tobramycin versus gentamicin in combination with vancomycin and nystatin for alimentary tract suppression in leukemia patients. *Eur J Cancer* 15:35-44, 1979.
23. Gurwith, M. J., Brunton, H. L., Lank, B. A., et al. A prospective controlled investigation of prophylactic trimethoprim-sulfamethoxazole in hospitalized granulocytopenic patients. *Am J Med* 66:248-256, 1979.
24. Dekker, A. W., Rozenberg-Arska, M., Sixma, J. J., et al. Prevention of infection by trimethoprim-sulfamethoxazole plus amphotericin B in patients with acute nonlymphoblastic leukemia. *Ann Intern Med* 95:555-559, 1981.

25. Pizzo, P. A., Robichaud, J., Brenda, K. E., *et al.* Oral antibiotic prophylaxis in patients with cancer. A double-blind randomized placebo-controlled trial. *J Pediatr* 102:125-133, 1983.
26. Bauernfeind, A., and Petermiller, C. *In vitro* activity of ciprofloxacin, norfloxacin and nalidixic acid. *Eur J Clin Microbiol* 2:111-115, 1983.
27. Hathorn, J. W., Rubin, M., and Pizzo, P. A. Empiric antibiotic therapy in febrile neutropenic cancer patients: Clinical efficacy and impact of monotherapy. *Antimicrob Agents Chemother* 31:971-977, 1987.
28. Alpen, E. L., and Sheline, G. E. Combined effects of thermal burn and whole body x-irradiation on survival time and mortality. *Ann Surg* 140:113-118, 1954.

Treatment of Infectious Complications
of the Hematopoietic Syndrome

Alexandre B. Oliveira

Introduction

From a strictly therapeutic point of view, bone marrow failure resulting from irradiation presents three main challenges to the clinician: (1) to correct any metabolic disturbances, either of the hydroelectrolytic compartment or of a nutritional nature; (2) to compensate for cytopenias, particularly of granulocytes and platelets; and (3) to prevent or treat infections. These goals can be achieved only through supportive, substitutive, or compensative therapies. In this chapter, I summarize the principal therapies that have been adopted for preventing and treating the infectious complications of the hematopoietic syndrome—complications that derive basically from transient granulocytopenia, which usually lasts for about 2 weeks. Severe bone marrow failure appears when significant body volumes receive doses of about 4-6 Gy within a short period of time. The clinician must bear in mind that the hematopoietic syndrome can put the life of an irradiated person at risk. Patients with severe granulocytopenia (less than $100/\mu L$) tend to develop early and possibly fatal infectious fevers. Despite the possibility that a concomitant hemorrhage might occur, which certainly would contribute to an increase in the mortality rate, it has seldom been observed in accidentally irradiated persons. Infectious complications are responsible for most fatalities. The basic rules adopted for preventing and treating infectious complications observed in accidentally irradiated persons do not differ substantially from those used for treating cancer patients who present granulocytopenia as a consequence of either the underlying disease or their chemotherapy or radiotherapy regimens.

Antibacterial Therapy

Previous investigations emphasized the importance of an early empirical antibiotic regimen for successful control of infection in granulocytopenic patients.

A. R. OLIVEIRA, Institudo Nuclebra de Seguridade Social, Av. Presidente Wilson, 231-8°, *Rio de Janeiro, Brazil, Cep.:20.030.*

Treatment of Radiation Injuries, Edited by
D. Browne *et al.*, Plenum Press, New York, 1990

To provide optimal antibiotic coverage against both gram-negative and gram-positive pathogens, it has become standard medical practice to associate two or even three antibiotics characterized by broad-spectrum coverage and adequate serum bactericidal activity. The most traditional and disseminated association is one that combines three groups of antimicrobial agents capable of countering organisms existing in immunocompromised patients.[1] This protocol includes an aminoglycoside group representative (gentamicin or amikacin), a first-generation cephalosporin (cephalotin), and an antipyocyanic, penicillinlike agent (carbenicillin, tobramycin, or piperacillin). This antibiotic regimen was used empirically on some irradiated persons in the New Jersey, Algeria, Chernobyl, and Goiânia accidents.[2]

Recently, National Cancer Institute (NCI) investigators reported results of trials, involving a significant number of cancer patients, that compared findings obtained either with a combined treatment (Keflin, gentamicin, and carbenicillin) or with third-generation cephalosporin (ceftazidime) alone. Investigators concluded that ceftazidime monotherapy performed better than the classical association.[3-5] The general rule for both antibiotic regimens is to maintain the course until the results of microbial studies indicate either that treatment should be continued or that changes are necessary to ensure more specific action against the pathogen.

Imipenem, a new beta-lactam antibiotic, seems to cover a broader spectrum of activity than the third-generation cephalosporins, acting not only on organisms responsive to ceftazidime but also against some coagulase-negative staphylococci, *Listeria*, enterococci, and a number of anaerobes. These qualities indicate that imipenem is a valid alternative to ceftazidime for monotherapy regimens on febrile granulocytopenic patients.[6]

Newly developed quinolones, among which oral norfloxacin is preeminent, have been used prophylactically to suppress the gastrointestinal (GI) tract colonization normally observed in patients with bone marrow failure who were treated previously with broad-spectrum antibacterial antibiotics.[7] One highly desirable effect of this therapy is the possibility of eradicating the pathogenic gram-negative bacterial flora and concomitantly preserving the anaerobic flora that could act as a barrier. In some centers, the use of oral norfloxacin drastically reduced the incidence of gram-negative sepsis in sterile chambers.

The efficacy of vancomycin seems to be well established in treating secondary infections by gram-positive pathogens, but only when clinical and microbial data suggest its use. A recent and extensive review concluded that this drug "need not be included in routine empirical therapy for febrile neutropenic patients."[8] On the other hand, its use would be advisable in hospitals whenever a high incidence of infections caused by *Staphylococcus aureus* and anaerobics was detected.

Prophylaxis of Endogenous Gastrointestinal Infections With Oral Antibiotics

The experience gained from treating both radiation accident victims and immunocompromised cancer patients suggests instituting oral antibiotic therapy to eliminate pathogens that are usually present in the GI tract, thereby avoiding the subsequent systemic bacterial invasion that has severe repercussions on granulocytopenic patients. The regimen adopted has been the combination of trimethoprim and sulfamethoxazole (TMP/SMX). Recent studies assessing the potential benefits of bacterial therapy with different types of absorbable and nonabsorbable antibiotics conclude, however, that information is insufficient to warrant using oral antibiotics routinely for granulocytopenic patients.[3]

Empirical Antifungal Therapy

It is well established that immunosuppressed patients have greater risk of developing fungal infections. The principal indicator for using antifungal therapy is the persistence of fever for 4 to 7 days in neutropenic patients receiving empirical broad-spectrum antibiotic therapy. Apparently, immunocompromised patients respond favorably if an early antifungal regimen is instituted to prevent the growth of fungi, which invariably occurs in neutropenic patients under broad-spectrum antibiotic coverage, and to prevent the systemic dissemination of subclinical infection. Randomized studies conducted at NCI involving three groups of patients demonstrated the efficacy of amphotericin B in treating high-risk immunocompromised patients.[3] Limitations on the use of this drug arise from its potential for toxic effects: chills, fever, anaphylactic reactions, and nephrotoxicity. Recently, with the advent of imidazole derivatives, such as ketoconazole, an efficacy similar to that of amphotericin B was obtained. Intraconazole seems to be even more effective than ketoconazole. The disadvantage of these agents is that they are absorbable only in an acid medium.

Treatment of Interstitial Pneumonia

The possibility of acute and diffuse interstitial pneumonia occurring in irradiated patients showing profound bone marrow failure was evidenced in the Chernobyl accident. When the pneumonia was related to rapid evolution in the clinical picture, the subsequent outcome was fatal. The Russian specialists, despite the lack of objective data, tended to associate the presence of interstitial pneumonitis in Chernobyl victims with the activation of cytomegalovirus. On the other hand, in granulocytopenic cancer patients, these pulmonary infiltrates are predominantly related to *Pneumocystis carinii*. Under such circumstances, the usual antibiotic coverage would be indicated, using TMP/SMX plus erythromycin with broad-spectrum antibacterial agents (ceftazidime or a conventional antibiotic regimen).[3]

Antiviral Therapy

Herpetic infection, one of the most frequent complications in granulocytopenic patients, can occasionally cause a serious therapeutic problem, mainly if there is dissemination to other organs. Now that antiviral drugs of relatively low toxicity are available for treating and preventing herpes virus, it is possible to reduce considerably the morbidity and mortality arising from viral infections. One of the most widely used drugs for preventing and treating herpetic lesions observed in immunosuppressed patients is acyclovir, which was used successfully in Chernobyl to treat herpes simplex lesions located on the face and on the labial and buccal mucosae. Viral skin lesions responded favorably to topical application of acyclovir ointment. In the Goiânia accident, eight patients received oral or intravenous acyclovir for antiviral prophylaxis. Other antiviral agents, such as viradabine and interferons, have been extensively investigated and have also been considered for use in these situations.[9]

Problems Related to the Use of In-Dwelling, Intravenous Central Catheters

Conventional catheters have shown little efficacy for patients requiring simultaneous perfusions for relatively long periods. Triple-lumen catheters (Multi-Med) have proved efficient not only with respect to their tolerance but also in relation to their long-term perviousness, permitting easier parenteral administration of fluids, blood compounds, and nutrients. However, one of the disadvantages of this technique is the appreciable development of infections. Some pathogens are directly implicated in the infections that derive from use of central access lines, such as gram-positive organisms (coagulase-negative *Staphylococcus*). The experience acquired in treating febrile neutropenic cancer patients advocates use of antibiotics (principally vancomycin) to complement the antibiotic regimen previously adopted, but only when there are clear signs of inflammation at the site of the catheter. Another practical question is what to do if an extending inflammatory process is detected along the subcutaneous tunneled path. In this situation, the only option available is to remove the device immediately. In the case of positive cultures for certain pathogens (*Bacillus* species and fungi), withdrawal of the catheter would also be indicated. Serial cultures of all catheter orifices are obviously required.[3]

Adjuvant Therapy for Infection in Bone Marrow Failure Caused by Accidental Radiation

To complement the antimicrobial action of the above-mentioned procedures, the literature dealing with infectious complications in granulocytopenic patients, particularly in those cases deriving from accidental exposure, mentions various therapeutic techniques: granulocyte transfusions, passive immunization, and colony-stimulating factors.

Granulocyte Transfusions

Despite the apparently rational explanation for using granulocyte transfusions, detailed observations of their actual efficacy have demonstrated no clear, unequivocal benefits to granulocytopenic patients. In addition to requiring sufficient and reliable supply routes, such transfusions present the adverse effects of alloimmunization, transfusion reactions, transmission of cytomegalovirus, and undesirable interaction with amphotericin B. Given the information available at present, there is no valid justification for using this procedure.[10]

Passive Immunization

In most immunosuppressed patients, one observes a substantial decrease in serum immunoglobulin levels, which theoretically could induce or facilitate the outbreak of infections. The use of immune gamma globulins could be efficacious not only in preventing but also in treating possible infections in neutropenic patients. High doses of gamma globulins were given intravenously to Chernobyl patients when fever persisted longer than 24 to 48 hours despite the extensive antibiotic coverage regimen instituted. Gamma globulins were also used in combination with amphotericin B. The potential clinical benefits of this technique must be better estimated for inclusion in future treatment protocols.

Colony-Stimulating Factors

Promising and exciting research involves the clinical application of colony-stimulating factors (CSF's) obtained through DNA recombinant techniques. One of these biosynthetically manufactured drugs, granulocyte-macrophage colony-stimulating factor (GM-CSF), was used on Goiânia patients with bone marrow failure, with the assumption that residual stem cells must exist.[11] A factor capable of stimulating residual stem cells to proliferate and differentiate might place many functionally immunocompetent cells in circulation rapidly and effectively, thus recomposing the natural human defense mechanisms. The duration of neutropenia was reduced, which, in principle, would reduce the risk of infection.

Also, some studies have shown GM-CSF to be effective in inhibiting neutrophil migration, increasing the antibody-dependent cellular toxicity, and augmenting phagocytosis capacity.[12,13]

References

1. Schimpff, S. C., Satterlee, W., Young, V. M., *et al.* Empiric therapy with carbenicillin and gentamicin for febrile patients with cancer and granulocytopenia. *N Eng J Med* 284:1061-1065, 1971.
2. Hubner, K. F., and Fry, S. A., Eds. *The Medical Basis for Radiation Accident Preparedness.* Elsevier North Holland, Inc., New York, 1980.
3. Rubin, M., Hathorn, J. W., and Pizzo, P. A. Controversies in the management of febrile neutropenic cancer patients. *Cancer Invest* 6(2):167-184, 1988.
4. Pizzo, P. A., Hathorn, J. W., Hiemenz, J., *et al.* A randomized trial comparing ceftazidime alone with combination antibiotic therapy in cancer patients with fever and neutropenia. *N Eng J Med* 315(9):552-558, 1986.
5. Dejace, P., and Klastersky, J. Comparative review of combination therapy: Two beta-lactams versus beta-lactam plus aminoglycoside. *Am J Med* 80(6B):29-38, 1986.
6. Wade, J. C., Standiford, H. C., Drusano, G. L., *et al.* Potential of imipenem as a single-agent empiric antibiotic therapy of febrile neutropenic patients with cancer. *Am J Med* 78(5A):62-72, 1985.
7. Karp, J. E., Merz, W. G., Hendricksen, C., *et al.* Oral norfloxacin for prevention of gram-negative bacterial infections in patients with acute leukemia and granulocytopenia. *Ann Intern Med* 106:1-7, 1987.
8. Rubin, M., Hathorn, J. W., Marshall, D., *et al.* Gram-positive infections and the use of vancomycin in 550 episodes of fever and neutropenia. *Ann Intern Med* 108:30-35, 1988.
9. Wong, K. K., and Hirsch, M. S. Herpes virus infections in patients with neoplastic diseases. Diagnosis and therapy. *Am J Med* 76:464-478, 1984.
10. Winston, D. J., Ho, W. G., and Gale, R. P. Therapeutic granulocyte transfusions for documented infections. *Ann Intern Med* 97:509-515, 1982.
11. Butturini, A., DeSouza, P. C., Gale, R. P., *et al.* Use of recombinant granulocyte-macrophage colony-stimulating factor in the Brazil radiation accident. *Lancet* II:471-475, 1988.
12. Grabstein, K. H., Urdal, D. L., Tushiaski, R. J., *et al.* Induction of macrophage tumoricidal activity by granulocyte-macrophage colony-stimulating factor. *Science* 232:506-508, 1986.
13. Weisbart, R. H., Golde, D. W., Clark, S. C., *et al.* Human granulocyte-macrophage colony-stimulating factor is a neutrophil activator. *Nature* 314:361-363, 1985.

Role of Immunotherapy in Preventing and Managing Postirradiation Infections

Richard I. Walker

Introduction

Infection is the single most important complication of otherwise survivable exposures to radiation. For example, in mice given an LD_{50} of radiation,[1] the animals that develop infections are the ones that die. These infections, which are often of enteric origin, are not seen in mice that survive the exposure.

Infection was a major cause of death in individuals seriously injured at Chernobyl, in Japan, and in other radiation accidents. The regimen used with Chernobyl victims reflected state-of-the-art treatment in controlling infections in immunocompromised individuals.

Persons with severe radiation exposures at Chernobyl were treated prophylactically with selective decontaminants—poorly absorbed antibiotics were used to restrict the bacteria that are opportunistic pathogens. These antibiotics, however, do not reduce the number of more benign anaerobic flora that contribute to intestinal resistance to colonization by other organisms.[2]

Temperature elevations in neutropenic patients from Chernobyl were treated empirically with two or three different antibiotics. If resolution was not obtained quickly, antifungal treatment was added. This approach was reasonably successful in patients with radiation injuries only, but it was less effective in patients with radiation-induced enteritis, graft-versus-host reactions, or combined injuries.

Basic surgical, supportive, and antimicrobial therapies will continue to be a cornerstone of treating victims of radiation and combined injuries (table 1). However, revolutionary new drugs that promise to extend postirradiation survival are becoming available. In recent years we have seen the development

R. I. WALKER, Infectious Diseases Department, Naval Medical Research Institute, Bethesda, Maryland 20814-5055.

Treatment of Radiation Injuries, Edited by
D. Browne *et al.*, Plenum Press, New York, 1990

Table 1. Approaches to Managing Sepsis
After Irradiation

Established approaches

- Wound debridement
- Topical antimicrobials and dressings
- Environmental control of nosocomials
- Minimal use of invasive and indwelling devices
- Fluid and electrolyte resuscitation
- Nutritional support
- Antibiotics and antimicrobial agents
- Pressor agents

New approaches

- Selective decontamination of gut
- Early administration of immunomodulators
  and/or hematopoietic modulators
- Growth factors
- Immunoglobulin G (antilipopolysaccharide)
- Antibody to tumor necrosis factor (cachectin)

---

of safer, biochemically defined immunomodulators and recombinantly produced growth factors and cytokines. Alone and in combination with each other and with conventional treatments, these immunoenhancing agents hold promise for major advances in the management of victims of irradiation and other trauma.

Enhancing Systemic Resistance to Microorganisms

Although granulocytes are reduced in number after exposure to radiation and concomitant increases in susceptibility to infection occur, macrophages remain and are at least partially functional. Enhancement of the macrophage antimicrobial activity can be a productive means of immunomodulation.

Immunomodulators

For years, various immunomodulating substances, often derived from microorganisms, have been used to enhance general resistance to infectious agents. Some of these agents from gram-negative bacteria, lipopolysaccharide, or endotoxin also regulate hematopoiesis. Unfortunately, many of these substances have toxic side effects. Newer agents now provide immunomodulation without significant side effects.

Some of the β-1,3 glucans from *Saccharomyces cerevisiae* have broad-spectrum benefits against infectious diseases.[3] Patchen *et al.*[4] showed that, in mice, 1.5 mg of glucan given 1 hour after radiation exposure enhances not only hematopoietic recovery but also host resistance to opportunistic infections that occur before significant hematopoietic regeneration takes place. This early enhanced resistance to microbial invasion in glucan-treated irradiated mice could be correlated with enhanced macrophage function.

Findings such as by Patchen et al.[4] have significant implications not only for therapy of radiation injury but also for the use of radioprotectors. The potential of immunomodulating substances can be increased after exposure to radiation as cells are protected from initial radiation injury. For example, WR-2721 can be used at a relatively safe dose (200 mg/kg) 30 minutes before exposure to radiation if glucan (250 mg/kg) is given 1 hour after radiation.[5] When WR-2721 and glucan are used together, radiation resistance (as shown by survival) is much greater than when either substance is used alone.

Monophosphoryl lipid A (MPL; obtained by chemical modification of toxic lipid A from heptoseless Re mutants of *Salmonella* species) and trehalose dimycolate (TDM; a cell wall glycolipid produced by *Mycobacteria, Nocardiae,* and *Corynebacteriae*) protected mice from radiation-induced lethality when given before or shortly after exposure.[6] Like glucan, MPL and TDM can enhance nonspecific resistance to infection. When mice given a sublethal exposure to cobalt-60 (7 Gy) were treated 1 hour after exposure and then challenged 4 days later with *Klebsiella pneumoniae,* a high percentage of those treated with an MPL-TDM mixture (figure 1; G. Madonna, unpublished data) or glucan survived, but all mice given saline died.

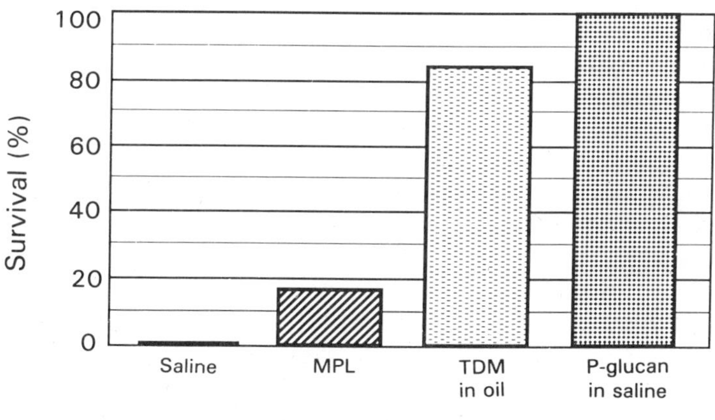

Figure 1. Survival of mice infected with *Klebsiella pneumoniae* 4 days after 7 Gy of cobalt-60 radiation. No saline-treated animals survived, but mice treated with (1) monophosphoryl lipid A (MPL) and trehalose dimycolate (TDM) and (2) particulate (P) glucan were significantly protected against death if given the immunomodulators 1 hour after exposure to radiation.

Experiments in which mice were exposed to 10.25 Gy of cobalt-60 and administered either TDM or saline 1 hour after irradiation show that TDM reduces naturally occurring postirradiation infections.[6] At intervals, livers were homogenized and cultured for bacteria. At 1, 3, and 5 days after irradiation, no bacteria were isolated from livers in either group. On days 7, 9, and 11, 20 to 40 bacteria were isolated from livers of TDM-treated mice, whereas the number of bacteria isolated from livers of saline-treated mice increased from 50 on day 7 to 3,000 on day 11. These data suggest that bacteria are still translocating from the intestine but that systemic defenses are enhanced in the TDM-treated animals.

Combined Injury

Comparing mortality of germ-free and conventional mice undergoing irradiation or irradiation and wounding shows that combined injury is also complicated by infections.[7] Germ-free mice can survive a radiation dose that kills half the conventional animals. Mortality in conventional animals is increased to 100 percent if a 3-cm dermal wound is superimposed on the radiation injury, but only a minimal number (17 percent) of germ-free animals succumb.

Immunotherapy of combined injury may be more difficult than treatment of radiation injury alone, as was seen with patients at Chernobyl and in mice treated with TDM after irradiation and wounding (G. Madonna, unpublished data). In contrast to mice that were only irradiated and given TDM, animals with combined injury died much sooner, and the TDM did not extend survival.

Multiple Treatment Interventions

Multiple treatment interventions may be necessary in severely immunocompromised individuals, such as those with combined injury. For example, sublethally irradiated mice given 10 $LD_{50/30}$ K. pneumoniae were well protected as measured by survival if treated with TDM.[6] This protection was not detected if the animals were challenged with 5,000 $LD_{50/30}$ K. pneumoniae. However, if the mice were treated once daily for 10 days with ceftriaxone therapy (75 mg/kg) in addition to TDM treatment, protection with the immunomodulator was again detectable.

Similarly, a synergistic effect on survival was found in irradiated mice given both pefloxacin and glucan (I. Brook, personal communication). In these experiments, 95-percent survival was obtained when the treatments were administered together, compared to 20-percent to 40-percent survival when each of the agents was administered alone.

Cytokines and Growth Factors

Immunomodulators activate macrophages that subsequently release mediators, including growth factors and cytokines. These factors can substitute for the immunomodulators in many cases, because they not only promote hematopoiesis but also enhance the function of mature cells. For example, interleukin-1, human granulocyte colony-stimulating factor, and small amounts of tumor necrosis factor (TNF) enhance nonspecific resistance to infection.[8-10]

Excessive quantities of TNF initiate the symptoms of septic shock. Another form of immunotherapy has been reported, in which monoclonal antibodies to TNF were used to prevent septic shock in baboons during lethal bacteremia.[11] This type of passive immunotherapy deserves further evaluation in hosts in which serious infections occur.

Immunotherapy of Mucosal Barriers to Infection

The intestinal lumen contains many bacteria, and presents a major source of infection after irradiation. Numerous factors (i.e., peristalsis, mucus, and colonization resistance) control populations of bacteria in the normal intestine, but many of these controls are lost after irradiation, as in the case of TNF indigenous segmented microflora.[12] As these and probably other relatively benign flora are lost, facultatively anaerobic flora increase in number until lethal infection occurs.

Sepsis is not a major problem when radiation doses produce the gastro-intestinal syndrome. However, with lower doses of radiation, death is caused by infection as a result of deficits in both hematopoietic status and intestinal barriers. One barrier that may be enhanced with immunotherapy is the lymphoepithelial system, as seen in the Peyer's patches.

The lymphoepithelial system is made up of normal intestinal epithelial cells, modified epithelial cells called M-cells, and associated macrophages and lymphocytes.[13] M-cells have short, irregular microvilli (microfolds) and derive directly from undifferentiated crypt cells. They have thin cytoplasmic extensions surrounding lymphoreticular cells. Most importantly, these cells are actively pinocytotic and endocytotic and, therefore, act as antigen-sampling structures. Macrophages are seen in association with lymphocyte clusters beneath the M-cells, where they are involved in defense and immunologic responses to microorganisms and other antigens passed through the M-cells.

It may be possible to increase antimicrobial activity of Peyer's patch macrophages by using immunomodulators. This possibility is indicated by inducing increases in the numbers of these cells in mouse Peyer's patches by oral administration of *Listeria monocytogenes*.[14] These animals were then able to restrict growth of *Salmonella enteritidis*, a mouse pathogen, at the mucosal site. This approach to immunotherapy may be of major importance, because the Peyer's patch M-cell is becoming recognized as an important portal of entry for numerous pathogens in normal animals,[15-19] and it could also facilitate translocation of increasing numbers of opportunistic pathogens in immunosuppressed individuals with defective lymphoreticular systems.

In areas of the intestine where Peyer's patches are not found, intestinal phagocytes could be responsible for translocation of bacteria. Wells *et al.* showed that when beads of various colors are placed in different ligated intestinal loops, macrophages that subsequently are found in the mesenteric lymph nodes contain beads of only one color.[20,21] This finding suggests that macrophages transport the beads from the loop.

Conclusion

Opportunistic pathogens may exploit the M-cell or macrophage route to leave the intestine. In the future, this source of life-threatening infection may be blocked by using immunomodulators and cytokines to augment the antibacterial activity of surviving cells and to replenish cells lost because of injury. Microspheres (J. Eldridge, personal communication) are now available, for example, that may be used to deliver immunotherapeutic agents to the Peyer's patches and macrophages of the mucosal barrier. As these approaches are developed in the future, it may become possible to enhance not only systemic defenses but also mucosal defenses, thereby further reducing infectious complications significantly.

References

1. Miller, C. P., Hammond, C. W., and Tompkins, M. The incidence of bacteria in mice subjected to whole-body x-radiation. *Science* 3:540-551, 1950.
2. van der Waaij, D., Berghuis-de Vries, J. M., and Lekkerkerk-van der Wees, J. E. C. Colonization resistance of the digestive tract and spread of bacteria to the lymphatic organs of mice. *J Hyg* 70:335-342, 1972.
3. Song, M., and DiLuzio, N. R. Yeast glucan and immunotherapy of infectious diseases. In: *Lysosomes in Applied Biology.* J. T. Dingle, P. J. Jacques, and I. H. Shaw, Eds. Elsevier North Holland, Amsterdam, 1979, pp. 533-547.
4. Patchen, M. L., D'Alesandro, M. M., Brook, I., *et al.* Glucan: Mechanisms involved in its "radioprotective" effect. *J Leukocyte Biol* 42:95-105, 1987.
5. Patchen, M. L., MacVittie, T. J., and Jackson, W. E. Postirradiation glucan administration enhances the radioprotective effects of WR-2721. *Radiat Res* 117:59-69, 1989.
6. Madonna, G. S., Ledney, G. D., Elliott, T. B., *et al.* Trehalose dimycolate enhances resistance to infection in neutropenic animals. *Infect Immun* 57:2495-2501, 1989.
7. Donati, R. M., McLaughlin, M. M., and Stromberg, L-W. R. Combined surgical and radiation injury. VIII. The effect of the gnotobiotic state on wound closure. *Experientia* 29:1388-1390, 1973.
8. Matsumoto, M., Matsubara, S., Matsuno, T., *et al.* Protective effect of human granulocyte colony-stimulating factor on microbial infection in neutropenic mice. *Infect Immun* 55:2715-2720, 1987.
9. Minami, A., Fujimoto, K., Ozaki, Y., *et al.* Augmentation of host resistance to microbial infections by recombinant human interleukin-1α. *Infect Immun* 56:3116-3120, 1988.

10. Nakane, A., Minagawa, T., and Kato, K. Endogenous tumor necrosis factor (cachectin) is essential to host resistance against *Listeria monocytogenes* infection. *Infect Immun* 56:2563-2569, 1988.

11. Tracey, K. J., Fong, Y., Hesse, D. G., et al. Anti-cachectin/TNF monoclonal antibodies prevent septic shock during lethal bacteremia. *Nature* 330:662-664, 1987.

12. Porvaznik, M., Walker, R. I., and Gillmore, J. D. Reduction of the indigenous filamentous microorganisms in rat ilea following gamma-radiation. *Scan Electron Microsc* 3:15-22, 1979.

13. Sneller, M. C., and Strober, W. M cells and host defense. *J Infect Dis* 154:737-741, 1986.

14. MacDonald, T. T., Bashore, M., and Carter, P. B. Nonspecific resistance to infection expressed within the Peyer's patches of the small intestine. *Infect Immun* 37:390-392, 1982.

15. Walker, R. I., Schmauder-Chock, E. A., Parker, J. L., et al. Selective association and transport of *Campylobacter jejuni* through M cells of rabbit Peyer's patches. *Can J Microbiol* 34:1142-1147, 1988.

16. Kohbata, S., Yokoyama, H., and Yabuuchi, E. Cytopathogenic effect of *Salmonella typhi* GI FU 10007 on M cells of murine ileal Peyer's patches in ligated ileal loops: An ultrastructural study. *Microbiol Immunol* 30:1225-1237, 1986.

17. Inman, L. R., and Cantey, J. R. Specific adherence of *Escherichia coli* (strain RDEC-1) to membranous (M) cells of the Peyer's patch in *Escherichia coli* diarrhea in the rabbit. *J Clin Invest* 71:1-8, 1983.

18. Owen, R. L., Pierce, N. F., Apple, R. J., et al. M cell transport of *Vibrio cholerae* from the intestinal lumen into Peyer's patches: A mechanism for antigen sampling and for microbial transepithelial migration. *J Infect Dis* 153:1108-1118, 1986.

19. Wassef, J. S., Keren, D. F., and Mailloux, J. L. Role of M cells in initial antigen uptake and in ulcer formation in the rabbit intestinal loop model of shigellosis. *Infect Immun* 57:858-863, 1988.

20. Wells, C. L., Maddaus, M. A., and Simmons, R. L. Proposed mechanisms for the translocation of intestinal bacteria. *Rev Infect Dis* 10:958-979, 1988.

21. Wells, C. L., Maddaus, M. A., Erlandsen, S. L., et al. Evidence for the phagocytic transport of intestinal particles in dogs and cats. *Infect Immun* 56:278-282, 1988.

Management of Fungal Infections Complicating Granulocytopenia

Implications for Patients With Radiation Injuries

Thomas J. Walsh and Philip A. Pizzo

Introduction

Invasive fungal infections are common complications reported with increasing frequency in granulocytopenic patients. These invasive mycoses cause substantial morbidity and mortality in patients receiving aggressive cytotoxic chemotherapy and ablative radiation therapy. The problem of invasive mycoses is further complicated by the appearance of new fungal pathogens and increasing reports of emerging resistance to established antifungal compounds. The two most common fungal groups infecting granulocytopenic patients are *Candida* species and *Aspergillus* species.

Portals of Entry

The alimentary tract is a site of considerable mucosal injury from exposure to radiation. Fungal infections of the alimentary tract of granulocytopenic patients (especially those due to *Candida* species) are the cause of significant discomfort, a deterrent to adequate nutrition, and a frequent portal of entry for systemic infection. Fungal infections of the alimentary tract may involve only the esophagus, stomach, or intestinal tract. More frequently, however, infection of the alimentary tract is an important portal of entry for systemic candidiasis, involving sites such as the liver, spleen, kidneys, heart, eyes, and brain. Intravenous catheters are the other major portal of entry for *Candida* species.

The respiratory tract is the major portal of entry for *Aspergillus* species. *Aspergillus* may cause locally invasive pneumonia or sinusitis. *Aspergillus* may disseminate from the lungs to cause lesions in the brain, kidney, liver, heart, and bones.

T. J. WALSH and P. A. PIZZO, Section of Infectious Diseases, Pediatric Branch, National Cancer Institute, Bethesda, Maryland 20892.

Treatment of Radiation Injuries, Edited by
D. Browne *et al.*, Plenum Press, New York, 1990

Classification

Most of the mycoses that complicate antineoplastic chemotherapy and radiation are nosocomial fungal infections. The nosocomial mycoses have been recently classified by Walsh and Pizzo[1] as either type 1 (hospital acquired) or type 2 (hospital associated). For example, most cases of nosocomial aspergillosis are type 1, while most cases of candidiasis are type 2 and arise from endogenous flora.

Causes of Oropharyngeal Candidiasis

Many studies have been conducted on the etiology, complications, and management of oropharyngeal candidiasis.[2-8] One such study by Meunier *et al.*[8] represents the typical spectrum of the *Candida* species that causes oropharyngeal candidiasis. The predominant organism is *C. albicans*; followed by *C. tropicalis* and then by other species, including *Torulopsis glabrata*; and finally by *C. parapsilosis*. Mixed infections due to these and other species are common.

Causes of Systemic Fungal Infection

The causes of systemic fungal infection include *C. albicans, C. tropicalis, C. parapsilosis, C. krusei, Aspergillus fumigatus, A. flavus, Trichosporon beigelii, Fusarium* species, and dematiacious fungi. Surveillance cultures are thought to be helpful in identifying the patients who will progress toward invasive mycoses.

Use of Surveillance Cultures

The role of fungal surveillance cultures and the timing of initiation of amphotericin-B therapy are two of the important and controversial issues of management of fungal infections in granulocytopenic patients. Sanford *et al.*[9] found that surveillance cultures for *Candida* and other fungi may serve as potential predictors of systemic fungal infections in granulocytopenic patients. Fungal surveillance cultures of urine, stool, and respiratory specimens were reviewed from 37 bone marrow transplant recipients and 52 patients with hematological malignancies. Among these patients, 67 percent were colonized by *C. albicans*, 28 percent by *C. tropicalis*, and none by *Aspergillus* species. There were 21 systemic fungal infections: 3 due to *C. albicans*, 16 due to *C. tropicalis*, and 2 due to *Aspergillus* species. The positive predictive value for patients colonized at one or more sites by *C. tropicalis* was 60 percent, but for *C. albicans* it was only 2 percent. By comparison, the negative predictive value of one or more surveillance cultures negative for *C. tropicalis* was 98 percent, and for *C. albicans*, 100 percent. Thus, the positive predictive value for *C. tropicalis* was good, but it was unreliable for *C. albicans*.

A subsequent study by Kramer *et al.*,[10] however, evaluated serial microbiological surveillance cultures in 271 patients with 652 episodes of fever and granulocytopenia. Because of the poor predictive value of surveillance cultures, these researchers could not justify the cost of routine fungal surveillance cultures in granulocytopenic patients. Other fungi have been identified as uncommon but emerging pathogens, including *Trichosporon* species. A study conducted by Walsh *et al.*[11] found that, among 15 patients colonized or infected by *Trichosporon* species, 4 of 5 patients (80 percent) with disseminated infection had negative surveillance cultures. Conversely, five colonized granulocytopenic patients did not develop active infection. Moreover, multiple cultures of the inanimate environment did not reveal *Trichosporon* species.

Several studies, however, have demonstrated the value of fungal cultures of the respiratory tract for early detection of pulmonary aspergillosis.[12-14] Aisner et al.[12] demonstrated that positive nasal surveillance cultures were predictive of the development of pulmonary aspergillosis during an ongoing outbreak of nosocomial aspergillosis in patients with hematological malignancies. In patients with positive nasal surveillance cultures, 10 of 11 acquired sinus or pulmonary aspergillosis, compared with 8 of 114 patients with negative nasal surveillance cultures who acquired aspergillosis. The predictive value of such surveillance has not been consistently corroborated by other institutions with different patient populations, environmental microbiology, and hospital epidemiology. Nevertheless, two studies, by Treger *et al.*[13] and Yu *et al.*,[14] have demonstrated the predictive value of lower respiratory tract cultures in high-risk granulocytopenic patients. However, these cultures are diagnostic cultures in high-risk patients and not surveillance cultures.

Empirical Antifungal Therapy

Because surveillance cultures and other diagnostic modalities had limited value for early recognition of the common invasive mycoses, and because delays in diagnosis were associated with high mortality, Pizzo et al.[15] studied the role of empirical antifungal therapy in cancer patients with prolonged fever and granulocytopenia. Among 652 episodes of fever and granulocytopenia in 271 patients, those with persistent fever and granulocytopenia were randomized to one of three groups: (1) discontinuation of antibiotics, (2) continuation of antibiotics, and (3) continuation of antibiotics with amphotericin B. Among those patients discontinuing antibiotics, six sustained bacterial sepsis. Among those continuing to receive antibiotics, 5 of 16 developed fungal infections, compared to 1 of 18 who continued to receive antibiotics and also received amphotericin B. Empirical antifungal therapy reduced the development of invasive fungal infections in high-risk patients. Several nonrandomized studies have continued to corroborate the value of empirical antifungal therapy in granulocytopenic patients. Data from the National

Cancer Institute (NCI) indicate that the frequency of fatal fungal infections has declined since the use of empirical amphotericin B. The early empirical use of amphotericin B in persistently or recurrently febrile granulocytopenic patients may prevent the development of some of the complications of invasive mycoses. Such complications include hepatosplenic candidiasis, pulmonary hemorrhage, and aspergillosis of the central nervous system.[16-18] Thus, patients with recurrent or persistent fever on or after day 7 of antibiotics at the NCI receive 0.5 mg/kg/day of empirical amphotericin B.

Treatment of Fungal Infections

For patients with documented established fungal infections, including disseminated candidiasis and pulmonary aspergillosis, the use of 0.5 mg/kg/day of amphotericin B may be inadequate. Higher doses of 1.0 to 1.5 mg/kg/day may be more effective against pulmonary aspergillosis and disseminated candidiasis in persistently granulocytopenic patients.[19,20] The addition of flucytosine may be beneficial in cases of renal candidiasis, hepatosplenic candidiasis, or central nervous system candidiasis. The combination of amphotericin B plus flucytosine versus high doses of amphotericin B in cases of pulmonary aspergillosis requires further investigation. More detailed discussions of the management of systemic mycoses in granulocytopenic patients may be found elsewhere.[21]

Conclusion

The early diagnosis of systemic mycoses in granulocytopenic patients is important; however, the ability to diagnose these infections remains limited. An empirical approach to antifungal therapy in high-risk granulocytopenic patients permits early treatment of invasive mycoses and may decrease the complications associated with these infections. These findings, obtained in the management of fungal infections in patients with therapeutically induced granulocytopenia, should be directly applicable to patients with radiation-induced granulocytes.

References

1. Walsh, T. J., and Pizzo, P. A. Nosocomial fungal infections. *Annu Rev Microbiol* 42:517-545, 1988.
2. Epstein, J., Truelove, E., and Izutzu, K. Oral candidiasis: Pathogenesis and host defense. *Rev Infect Dis* 6:96-106, 1984.
3. Holst, E. Natamycin and nystatin for treatment of oral candidiasis during and after radiotherapy. *J Prosthet Dent* 51:226-231, 1984.
4. Quintiliani, R., Owens, N. J., Quercia, R., et al. Treatment and prevention of oropharyngeal candidiasis. *Am J Med* 77(4D):44-48, 1984.

5. Rodu, B., Griffin, I., and Gockerman, J. Oral candidiasis in cancer patients. *South Med J* 77:312-314, 1984.
6. Walsh, T. J., and Grey, W. *Candida* epiglottitis in immunocompromised patients. *Chest* 9:482-485, 1987.
7. Schechtman, S., Fumaro, L., Robin, T., *et al.* Clotrimazole treatment of oral candidiasis in patients with neoplastic disease. *Am J Med* 76:91-94, 1984.
8. Meunier, F., Gerain, J., Snoeck, R., *et al.* Fluconazole therapy of oropharyngeal candidiasis in cancer patients. In: *Recent Trends in the Discovery, Development, and Evaluation of Antifungal Agents.* R. Fromtling, Ed. R. J. Prous Science, Barcelona, Spain, 1988, pp. 169-174.
9. Sanford, G. R., Merz, W. G., Wingard, J. R., *et al.* The value of fungal surveillance cultures as predictors of systemic fungal infections. *J Infect Dis* 142:503-509, 1980.
10. Kramer, B. S., Pizzo, P. A., Robichaud, K. J., *et al.* Role of serial microbiologic surveillance and clinical evaluation in the management of cancer patients with fever and granulocytopenia. *Am J Med* 72:561-568, 1982.
11. Walsh, T. J., Newman, K. R., Moody, M., *et al.* Trichosporonosis in patients with neoplastic disease. *Medicine (Baltimore)* 65:268-279, 1986.
12. Aisner, J., Murillo, J., Schimpff, S. C., *et al.* Invasive aspergillosis in acute leukemia: Correlation with nose cultures and antibiotic use. *Ann Intern Med* 90:4-9, 1979.
13. Treger, T. R., Visscher, D. W., Bartlett, M. S., *et al.* Diagnosis of pulmonary infection caused by *Aspergillus*: Usefulness of respiratory cultures. *J Infect Dis* 152:572-576, 1975.
14. Yu, V. L., Muder, R. R., and Poosattar, A. Significance of isolation of *Aspergillus* from the respiratory tract in diagnosis of invasive pulmonary aspergillosis. *Am J Med* 81:249-254, 1986.
15. Pizzo, P. A., Robichaud, K. J., Gill, F. A., *et al.* Empiric antibiotic and antifungal therapy for cancer patients with prolonged fever and granulocytopenia. *Am J Med* 72:101-110, 1982.
16. Thaler, M., Pastakia, B., Shawker, T. H., *et al.* Hepatic candidiasis in cancer patients: The evolving picture of the syndrome. *Ann Intern Med* 108:88-100, 1988.
17. Panos, R. J., Barr, L. F., Walsh, T. J., *et al.* Factors associated with fatal hemoptysis in cancer patients. *Chest* 94:1008-1013, 1988.
18. Walsh, T. J., Caplan, L. R., and Hier, D. B. *Aspergillus* infections of the central nervous system: A clinicopathological analysis. *Ann Neurol* 18:574-582, 1985.
19. Burch, P. A., Karp, J. B., and Merz, W. G. Favorable outcome of invasive *Aspergillus* in patients with acute leukemia. *J Clin Oncol* 5:1985-1993, 1987.
20. Horn, R., Wong, B., Koehn, T. B., *et al.* Fungemia in a cancer hospital: Changing frequency, earlier onset, and results of therapy. *Rev Infect Dis* 7:646-655, 1985.
21. Walsh, T. J., and Pizzo, P. A. Treatment of systemic fungal infections: Recent progress and current problems. *Eur J Clin Microbiol* 7:460-475, 1988.

Prevention of Infection With Endogenous Organisms

Gary P. Zaloga

Introduction

Infection is a major cause of organ failure and death in patients after radiation injury. Because most infections result from invasion by endogenous organisms from the gut and respiratory tract, in this chapter I discuss state-of-the-art methods for minimizing infections from these two sites.

Maintaining or Improving Gut Barrier Function

The gut mucosa normally serves as a barrier between luminal microorganisms and tissues. Invasion is prevented by mucosal secretions; a thick, villous structure with tight junctions between individual epithelial cells; luminal IgA (secreted primarily in bile); gut lymphocytic structures (i.e., Peyer's patches); and circulating immune cells (i.e., B- and T-lymphocytes and granulocytes).

Gut Growth Factors

Maintenance of gut structure and function depends on the constant supply of nutrients and growth factors in the gut lumen. Although the gut can receive these substances from both the gut lumen and the bloodstream, the luminal presence of nutrients and growth factors in the form of enteral nutrition is more effective in maintaining the gut than nutrients supplied through parenteral routes. Gut growth is stimulated by long-chain fatty acids, short-chain fatty acids produced by bacterial fermentation of carbohydrate in the gut lumen,[1,2] ketones, glucose, glutamine,[3-6] and polyamines.[7] Other trophic stimuli for the gut that result from enteral feeding include pancreatic and biliary secretions, endocrine factors (i.e., glucagon and gastrin), paracrine factors, neural factors, and increases in intestinal blood flow.

G. P. ZALOGA, Department of Anesthesia (Critical Care) and Medicine, Bowman Gray School of Medicine, Wake Forest University, Winston-Salem, North Carolina 27103.

Treatment of Radiation Injuries, Edited by
D. Browne *et al.*, Plenum Press, New York, 1990

Gut mucosal atrophy, a predilection for bacterial and fungal invasion, and increased mortality have been associated with the lack of enteral nutrition (i.e., use of either total parenteral nutrition (TPN) or no nutrition).[8-10] The epithelium of the gastrointestinal (GI) tract is a rapidly renewing tissue profoundly affected by food deprivation and starvation. During food deprivation, villus height and epithelial cell proliferation in the crypts decrease, cell migration up the villi slows, and overall mass (i.e., DNA content and protein content) of the intestinal wall is reduced. Disaccharidase activity in the brush border diminishes, and the capacity to digest protein and fat decreases. In addition, mucosal permeability increases,[11] and there is a loss of protective mucosal secretions. All of these factors predispose the host to invasion by microorganisms. Refeeding the gut (enteral nutrition) in unstressed individuals is associated with return of structure and function within 3 to 6 days. During this time, there is frequently a period of malabsorption while intestinal cells are being repleted.

Gut Bacterial Translocation

Gut-origin septic states (i.e., from bacterial or toxin translocation) may result from GI malnutrition (i.e., lack of enteral nutrition), gut bacterial overgrowth, loss of systemic immunity,[12,13] or loss of intestinal integrity due to colitis, radiation damage, chemotherapy, or hypoperfusion.[14,15] Bacteria and/or their toxins enter the portal circulation, activate macrophages and other immune cells, and cause the release of cytokines that damage organs, suppress the immune response, produce the septic state, and result in death.

Bacteremia from gut bacteria has been demonstrated in animals after hemorrhage[16] and is thought to contribute to sepsis and organ failure. Baker et al.[17] demonstrated translocation of bacteria from the gut to mesenteric lymph nodes, livers, and spleens of rats subjected to hemorrhagic shock. Rats subjected to 90 minutes of shock exhibited a greater degree of bacterial translocation than rats subjected to 30 or 60 minutes of shock. Many of these animals did not have positive blood cultures (which were obtained from the systemic venous circulation). Presumably, many bacteria fail to enter the systemic circulation because they are removed by the mesenteric lymph nodes and liver. It is also possible that organ damage is caused by endotoxin entry and not by viable bacteria. Sori et al.[18] radiolabeled *Escherichia coli*, fed them to rats, and then subjected the rats to hemorrhagic shock. Presence of radiolabeled bacteria in the blood following hemorrhage predicted mortality. Increased resistance to hemorrhagic shock and improved survival have been noted in cecectomized germ-free rats.[19] In addition, we have found that gut protection with enteral nutrition protects animals from liver damage during hemorrhage, presumably by preventing bacterial translocation.[20]

Bacterial translocation from the gut to the mesenteric lymph nodes and liver also has been demonstrated after trauma and burn injury.[21-24] Howerton and

Kolmen[23] labeled *Pseudomonas aeruginosa* organisms with fluorescein and fed them intragastrically to rats. Two days later one group of rats received a third-degree burn injury. Unburned rats did not develop bacteremia or culture-positive mesenteric lymph nodes. Burned rats developed bacteremia and culture-positive mesenteric lymph nodes with the fluorescein-labeled bacteria. Labeled *Pseudomonas* also was found deep in the burn wound. Gut blood flow decreased after burn injury, and the reduction was also associated with translocation of orally administered *Candida albicans* to the mesenteric lymph nodes.[25,26] Administration of enteral nutrition soon after burn injury improved intestinal blood flow and decreased the translocation of *C. albicans*.

Bacterial translocation from the gut is promoted when the immune defenses are impaired because of chemotherapy in athymic mice.[12,13,24,27] Chemical, chemotherapy, and radiation injury to the gut mucosa also promote bacterial/toxin translocation.[6,14,28] Bounous *et al.* have shown that elemental diets protect the intestinal epithelium from damage by 5-fluorouracil (5-FU) in rats[29] and humans.[30]

There is abundant clinical information suggesting that microorganisms translocate from the gut into the systemic circulation in humans. Stone *et al.*[31] have incriminated the gut as the source for systemic *Candida* infections, while others[32,33] have done so for bacteremia in septic surgical patients. The gut also has been implicated as the source of systemic and wound infection in immunocompromised, cancer, burn, and traumatized patients.

Enteral Nutrition Versus Total Parenteral Nutrition

Kudsk compared enteral feeding to TPN in well-nourished and malnourished animals with hemoglobin-*E. coli* peritonitis.[8,9] Enterally fed animals had improved survival (70 percent versus 38 percent for malnourished animals, 60 percent versus 20 percent for well-nourished animals). These and other data[10,11] suggest that host defenses (i.e., immunocompetence) are better when feeding occurs via the GI tract than through intravenous routes.

Renk *et al.*[34] measured lymphocyte responses in animals that had sustained femoral fractures. All animals had a depression in lymphocyte responses after injury, but lymphocyte responses recovered within 1 week in orally fed animals but not in intravenously fed animals. In a subsequent study,[35] lymphocyte responses to lipopolysaccharide and concanavalin A remained normal in enterally fed animals but became depressed in intravenously fed animals. In addition, biliary secretion of IgA has been shown to decrease in rats after intravenous feeding but not after enteral feeding.[36]

Alverdy *et al.*[37] studied the effect of an oral diet of standard rat chow, an elemental oral diet of TPN solution, and TPN on bacterial translocation from the gut in rats. Animals were fed each diet for 2 weeks, and then the mesenteric lymph nodes and cecum were removed and cultured. Two-thirds of animals fed TPN (18 of 27) had culture-positive mesenteric lymph nodes, compared with one-third (9 of 27) fed the oral elemental formula and none (of 30) fed the standard diet. There was also a significant increase in cecal bacterial counts in the TPN and oral elemental diet groups. These data suggest that parenteral nutrition and oral elemental diets promote bacterial translocation from the gut.

Border *et al.*[38] retrospectively examined the effect of enteral feeding on sepsis as measured by a septic severity score (SSS) in 66 patients admitted to the intensive care unit. The SSS is based on 16 measurements, including electrolytes, blood gases, inspired oxygen, positive-end expiratory pressure, leukocyte count, highest daily temperature, bilirubin, creatinine, platelets, and blood glucose. Only increased enteral protein intake was associated with a reduction in SSS and reduced bacterial evidence of sepsis. Patients who received almost twice as much protein parenterally as the patients who received protein enterally developed a higher SSS than enterally fed patients.

Studies also have demonstrated a reduction in sepsis with enteral nutrition. Alexander *et al.*[39] and Antonacci *et al.*[40] have shown that enteral nutrition is associated with reduced mortality and sepsis after burns. Alexander *et al.*[39] also demonstrated improved neutrophil opsonic function in burn patients receiving enteral alimentation, compared with parenteral nutrition. Moore[41] studied a group of patients undergoing laparotomy after trauma and randomized them to enteral feeding (n = 20) versus TPN (n = 23). The TPN group had higher overall morbidity and more infections (sepsis, abscess, and pneumonia). These data support the premise that enteral feeding in the postoperative period is more advantageous than TPN in protecting the gut barrier and preventing infections. Peterson *et al.*[42] also found that enteral nutrition reduced the incidence of sepsis in a group of trauma patients randomized to enteral feeding versus TPN.

Early Enteral Feeding

Early enteral feeding (within 12 hours of injury) also may benefit the organism by blunting the hypermetabolic response to critical illness.[25,43-45] This attenuation of hypercatabolism preserves lean body mass and can help preserve hepatic protein synthesis, respiratory muscle strength, and cardiac contractility. Administration of only Ringer's solution for the first 24 hours after burn injury has been associated with a 30-percent reduction in jejunal mucosal thickness and a 50-percent reduction in jejunal mucosal weight.[25] Feeding of an equivalent volume of a well-balanced enteral diet resulted in no loss of mucosal mass or thickness. Moore and Jones[46] studied 75 patients who were undergoing emergent celiotomy after abdominal trauma. The patients were randomized to early enteral feeding (within 12 to 18 hours of admission) or control diet (5 percent dextrose and water) for 5 days, followed by enteral feeding and supplemental TPN if needed. Septic morbidity was significantly greater in the control group. It was concluded that early enteral nutrition reduced the septic morbidity that follows major trauma.

Antacids, Gastrointestinal Bleeding, and Pneumonia

Stress ulcers were a major cause of morbidity and mortality in critically ill patients in the 1960's. Controlled studies demonstrated a reduction in gastric bleeding with antacids and histamine-2 (H2) receptor antagonists. However, in some studies of stress ulcer prophylaxis, the mortality in the placebo groups was lower than that in the patients receiving antacids or H2 blockers.[47,48]

Bacterial growth in the stomach occurs when the pH of gastric juices exceeds 3.5-4.0.[49-56] Use of antacids and H2 antagonists to neutralize acid has been implicated as a cause of nosocomial pneumonia,[49,50,52,54-59] a leading cause of death in hospitalized patients. It is usually caused by gram-negative bacilli, and frequently results from aspiration of bacteria from the oropharynx and stomach.[52-56,59,60]

Sucralfate (a cytoprotective, nonabsorbable agent with minimal acid-neutralizing capacity) is as efficacious as antacids and H2 blockers in preventing stress bleeding.[52,61,62] Use of sucralfate has been associated with a lower incidence of gastric colonization, tracheal colonization, pneumonia, and death, compared with antacids and H2 blockers.[52,56,61,63,64] Driks et al.[52] reported a 11.5-percent incidence of pneumonia in critically ill, intubated patients receiving sucralfate versus a 23.2-percent incidence in an antacid-H2 blocker group. Mortality was also lower in the sucralfate group (29.5 percent versus 46.4 percent).[52] Tryba[61] reported a 10-percent incidence of pneumonia in patients treated with sucralfate and a 34-percent incidence in patients treated with antacids.

Pirenzepine (an anticholinergic agent) also is effective in preventing stress bleeding. Like sucralfate, it is associated with a lower incidence of pneumonia, compared with antacids and H2 blockers.[56,57] These data suggest that agents that elevate gastric pH (i.e., eliminate the gastric acid barrier) increase the risk of nosocomial pneumonia and death by promoting gastric bacterial colonization.

Enteral Nutrition

The previous discussion indicates that enteral nutrition can protect gut structure and function, minimize bacterial translocation, and improve outcome in critically ill patients. The tolerance and benefits of enteral feeding depend upon the protein component used and the technique of administration.

Protein

Protein is better absorbed in peptide form than in free amino acid form[65-67] because specific transport systems exist in the small intestine for free amino acids, dipeptides, and tripeptides. Animals gain weight more quickly when fed protein hydrolysates, compared with intact protein and free amino acid-based enteral formulas. Absorption of amino acids is reduced in protein- or calorie-deprived patients, in critically ill patients, and in patients receiving only parenteral nutrition. In these patients, absorption of peptides is maintained or enhanced.[68-73] Peptide-based enteral feeding products stimulate absorption in the gut and reduce the incidence of diarrhea in critically ill patients and those with radiation enteritis.[66,68-73] Peptide-based enteral nutrition also produces better anabolic responses than intact protein diets,[71] and reduces nitrogen losses in the urine.[74] Some of the benefits of peptide enteral feedings result from the enhanced release of gut-trophic hormones, such as glucagon.[75] In addition, liquid diets containing crystalline amino acids increase the number of facultative enteric bacilli (i.e., *E. coli*) in the gut.[76,77] This increase in gut flora may predispose to bacterial translocation. The fecal flora are not altered with more complex diets. These observations suggest that peptides are better sources of nitrogen than free amino acids or intact proteins during refeeding in malnourished or critically ill patients.

Radiation Enteropathy

Radiation enteropathy (abdominal cramps with severe diarrhea) occurs in about one-third of adult patients and 70 percent of children undergoing intensive abdominal or pelvic irradiation.[68] Radiation enteropathy is associated with villus atrophy, loss of mucosal mucous, and loss of digestive enzymes. Walker *et al.*[28] noted the appearance of endotoxin and bacteria in the livers of mice after 8.5 Gy of total-body irradiation, suggesting increased translocation or decreased hepatic clearance.

Animals fed a casein-hydrolysate or elemental diet before and after irradiation are more likely to survive and lose less weight than animals eating regular food or intact protein formula.[69] Initial radiation damage to the intestine is not prevented, but recovery appears to be faster. With the prophylactic use of protein-hydrolysate or free amino acid feedings,[68,78] compared with normal diets (intact protein), improved weight gain, higher serum protein levels, and less diarrhea also are found in patients undergoing abdominal radiation. When given before and during irradiation, protein hydrolysates also preserve small bowel mucosa.[68] Both protein hydrolysates and free amino acid diets are effective in treating patients with established radiation enteropathy. Fecal fluid loss and energy losses are decreased in patients receiving these diets, compared with normal diets.[70] In addition, defined formula diets protect the intestinal epithelium from damage by 5-FU in rats[29] and humans.[30]

Techniques for Enteral Feeding

Enteral nutrition can be delivered by a variety of methods: oral, nasogastric, nasoduodenal, gastric (via gastrostomy), and jejunal (via feeding jejunostomy). The oral route is the easiest to use, is associated with the best gut preservation, and is the preferred route of nutrient administration in noncritically injured patients, especially if granulocytopenia is present. However, because many critically ill patients are anorexic and at risk for aspiration, the use of feeding tubes is necessary.

Gastric and colonic ileus are common in severely injured patients. However, the small intestine usually maintains good motility and absorption, even after multiple trauma, surgery, and burns. To determine whether patients who are critically ill with multiple trauma, respiratory failure, or sepsis could tolerate gastric feedings, we administered enteral nutrition via feeding tubes into the stomachs of 20 patients at a rate of 100 mL/hour. All patients developed large gastric residuals (> 150 mL) within 12 hours, indicative of poor gastric emptying. When switched to duodenal feedings, all patients tolerated the nutritional formulas without problems, indicating good small bowel function.

Aspiration of nutritional formulas and bacteria are also of concern when patients are fed gastrically. We monitored for aspiration by measuring tracheal glucose levels in patients receiving gastric or duodenal feedings. Six of 20 gastric-fed patients (30 percent) had an elevation in tracheal glucose concentration, while none of 20 patients fed via the duodenum had evidence of aspiration. These data indicate that duodenal feeding minimizes the risk of pulmonary aspiration.

Many clinicians place thin-bore weighted feeding tubes into the stomach, hoping that they will migrate spontaneously into the small bowel. We evaluated this technique in 100 critically ill patients and found that only 5 of 100 tubes passed spontaneously into the small intestine over a 3-day period. Metoclopramide had no effect on tube passage. Thus, we think that feeding tubes should be placed in the small intestine so that nutrition can be started as soon as possible after injury. We have been successful in placing feeding tubes in the duodenum using a corkscrew technique, i.e., a wire stylet is bent at a 30-degree angle just proximal to the distal tip of the tube, allowing for rotation of the tube through the pylorus. Tubes may also be placed in the duodenum by means of fluoroscopy or endoscopy.

Summary and Recommendations

These data suggest that enteral nutrition is superior to TPN. Enteral feeding, even in small quantities, should be introduced into the management program of patients as early as possible after injury—within 12 hours of admission for most patients. Early feeding is essential to help maintain gut mucosal structure and function, to blunt the hypermetabolic response to illness (i.e., reduce catabolic rate and minimize loss of lean muscle mass), to maintain immune function, to decrease the incidence of gut-origin sepsis, to maintain organ function (i.e., prevent progression to multiple-organ failure), to stimulate gut recovery, and to decrease mortality. Optimal enteral nutrition is best accomplished in critically ill patients with sterile, premixed enteral feeding formulas containing simple sugars (because disaccharidase activity may be low); small amounts of fermentable complex carbohydrates (to provide substrate for short-chain fatty acids); small peptides as the nitrogen source; and some long-chain fatty acids (for essential fatty acid repletion and as a gut-trophic stimulus). Enteral feeding may be advanced toward a normal diet once gut structure and function has returned to normal.

Because gastric emptying is frequently diminished in critically ill patients, and because gastric feedings may predispose to aspiration, we recommend continuous feeding into the small bowel by means of nasoduodenal tubes or jejunostomies. Less ill patients with intact gastric emptying may be able to tolerate oral or gastric nutrition. In immunocompromised patients, the oral route is preferable, provided adequate nutrition can be given.

When enteral nutrition cannot be given because the patient is incapable of oral intake, or it is deemed undesirable to place a thin-bore feeding tube (for example, there is a fear of mucosal ulceration in a severely granulocytopenic patient), patients should be started on parenteral nutrition. Gastric and tracheal colonization, pneumonia, and death may be minimized by using agents for stress ulcer prophylaxis that do not neutralize gastric pH (i.e., sucralfate).

References

1. Sakata, T., and von Engelhardt, W. Stimulatory effect of short chain fatty acids on the epithelial cell proliferation in rat large intestine. *Comp Biochem Physiol* 74A:459 (Abstract), 1983.
2. Rombeau, J. L., Rolandoelli, R. H., Kripke, S. A., *et al.* Experimental investigations of short-chain fatty acids as colonic fuels. In: *The Gastrointestinal Response to Injury, Starvation, and Enteral Nutrition.* 8th Ross Conference on Medical Research, Ross Laboratories, Columbus, Ohio, 1988, pp. 79-82.
3. Souba, W. W., Smith, R. J., and Wilmore, D. W. Glutamine metabolism by the intestinal tract. *JPEN* 9:608-617, 1985.
4. Hwang, T. L., O'Dwyer, S. T., Smith, R. J., *et al.* Preservation of small bowel mucosa using glutamine-enriched parenteral nutrition. *Surg Forum* 37:56-58, 1986.
5. Klimberg, V. S., Souba, W. W., Dolson, D., *et al.* Oral glutamine supports crypt cell turnover and accelerates intestinal healing following abdominal radiation. *JPEN* 13:11S (Abstract), 1989.
6. Fox, A. D., Kripke, S. A., DePaula, J., *et al.* Effect of a glutamine-supplemented enteral diet on methotrexate-induced enterocolitis. *JPEN* 12:325-331, 1988.
7. Dufour, C., Dandrifosse, G., Forget, P., *et al.* Spermine and spermidine induce intestinal maturation in the rat. *Gastroenterology* 95:112 (Abstract), 1988.

8. Kudsk, K. A., Carpenter, G., Peterson, S. R., *et al.* Effect of enteral and parenteral feeding in malnourished rats with hemoglobin-*E. coli* adjuvant peritonitis. *J Surg Res* 31:105-110, 1981.

9. Kudsk, K. A., Stone, J. M., Carpenter, G., *et al.* Enteral and parenteral feeding influences mortality after hemoglobin *E. coli* peritonitis in normal rats. *J Trauma* 23:605-609, 1983.

10. Peterson, S. R., Kudsk, K. A., Carpenter, G., *et al.* Malnutrition and immunocompetence: Increased mortality following an infectious challenge during hyperalimentation. *J Trauma* 21:528-533, 1981.

11. Rothman, D., Latham, M. C., and Walker, W. A. Transport of macromolecules in malnourished animals. I. Evidence of increased uptake of intestinal antigens. *Nutr Rev* 2:467-473, 1982.

12. Berg, R. D. Bacterial translocation from the gastrointestinal tracts of mice receiving immunosuppressive chemotherapeutic agents. *Curr Microbiol* 8:285-292, 1983.

13. Owens, W. E., and Berg, R. D. Bacterial translocation from the gastrointestinal tract of athymic (nu/nu) mice. *Infect Immun* 27:461-467, 1980.

14. Morehouse, J. L., Specian, R. D., Stewart, J. J., *et al.* Translocation of indigenous bacteria from the gastrointestinal tract of mice after oral ricinoleic acid treatment. *Gastroenterology* 91:673-682, 1986.

15. Brook, I., MacVittie, T. J., and Walker, R. I. Recovery of aerobic and anaerobic bacteria from irradiated mice. *Infect Immun* 46:270-271, 1984.

16. Koziol, J., Rush, B. F., Smith, S. M., *et al.* Occurrence of bacteremia during and after hemorrhagic shock. *J Trauma* 28:10-16, 1988.

17. Baker, J. W., Deitch, E. A., Berg, R. D., *et al.* Hemorrhagic shock induces bacterial translocation from the gut. *J Trauma* 28:896-906, 1988.

18. Sori, A. J., Rush, B. F., Lysz, T. W., *et al.* The gut as a source of sepsis after hemorrhagic shock. *Am J Surg* 155:187-192, 1988.

19. Heneghan, J. B., Peuler, M., Costrini, A., *et al.* Hemorrhagic shock in cecectomized germfree rats. *Surg Forum* 21:232-233, 1970.

20. Prielipp, R. C., Ward, K. A., and Zaloga, G. P. Peptide-based enteral nutrition prevents liver injury during severe hemorrhagic shock in rats. *Anesthesiology* 71:164 (Abstract), 1989.

21. Deitch, E. A., and Bridges, R. M. Effect of stress and trauma on bacterial translocation from the gut. *J Surg Res* 42:536-542, 1987.

22. Maejima, K., Deitch, E., and Berg, R. Promotion by burn stress of the translocation of bacteria from the gastrointestinal tracts of mice. *Arch Surg* 119:166-172, 1984.

23. Howerton, E. E., and Kolmen, S. N. The intestinal tract as a portal of entry of *Pseudomonas* in burned rats. *J Trauma* 12:335-340, 1972.

24. Deitch, E. A., Winterton, J., and Berg, R. Thermal injury promotes bacterial translocation from the gastrointestinal tract in mice with impaired T-cell-mediated immunity. *Arch Surg* 121:97-101, 1986.

25. Alexander, J. W. Influence of feeding route on metabolic response to injury. In: *The Gastrointestinal Response to Injury, Starvation, and Enteral Nutrition.* 8th Ross Conference on Medical Research, Ross Laboratories, Columbus, Ohio, 1988, pp. 41-42.

26. Inoue, S., Wirman, J. A., Alexander, J. W., *et al. Candida albicans* translocation across the gut mucosa following burn injury. *J Surg Res* 44:479-492, 1988.

27. Owens, W. E., and Berg, R. D. Bacterial translocation from the gastrointestinal tracts of thymectomized mice. *Curr Microbiol* 7:169-174, 1982.

28. Walker, R. I., Ledney, G. D., and Galley, C. B. Aseptic endotoxemia in radiation injury and graft-versus-host disease. *Radiat Res* 62:242-249, 1975.

29. Bounous, G., Hugon, J., and Gentile, J. M. Elemental diet in the management of the intestinal lesion produced by 5-fluorouracil in the rat. *Can J Surg* 14:298-311, 1971.

30. Bounous, G., Gentile, J. M., and Hugon, J. Elemental diet in the management of the intestinal lesion produced by 5-fluorouracil in man. *Can J Surg* 14:312-324, 1971.

31. Stone, H. H., Kolb, L. D., Currie, C. A., *et al. Candida* sepsis: Pathogenesis and principles of treatment. *Ann Surg* 179:697-711, 1974.

32. Fry, D. E., Flamer, T. W., Garrison, R. N., *et al.* Atypical clostridial bacteremia. *Surg Gynecol Obstet* 153:28-30, 1981.

33. Garrison, R. N., Fry, D. E., Berborich, S., *et al.* Enterococcal bacteremia: Clinical implications and determinants of death. *Ann Surg* 196:43-47, 1982.
34. Renk, C. M., Owens, D. R., Birkhahn, R. H., *et al.* Effect of intravenous or oral feeding on immunocompetence in traumatized rats. *JPEN* 4:587 (Abstract), 1985.
35. Birkhahn, R. H., and Renk, C. M. Immune response and leucine oxidation in oral and intravenous fed rats. *Am J Clin Nutr* 39:45-53, 1984.
36. Alverdy, J. C., Chi, H. S., and Sheldon, G. F. The effect of parenteral nutrition on gastrointestinal immunity: The importance of enteral stimulation. *Ann Surg* 202:681-684, 1985.
37. Alverdy, J. C., Aoys, E., and Moss, G. S. Total parenteral nutrition promotes bacterial translocation from the gut. *Surgery* 104:185-190, 1988.
38. Border, J., Hassett, J., LaDuca, J., *et al.* The gut origin septic states in blunt multiple trauma (ISS 40) in the ICU. *Ann Surg* 206:427-448, 1987.
39. Alexander, J. W., Macmillan, B. G., Stinnet, J. D., *et al.* Beneficial effects of aggressive protein feeding in severely burned children. *Ann Surg* 192:505-517, 1980.
40. Antonacci, A., Cowles, S., and Reaves, L. The role of nutrition in immunologic function. *Infect Surg* 3:590-602, 1984.
41. Moore, E. E. Early postinjury enteral feeding: Attenuated stress response and reduced sepsis. *Contemp Surgery* 32:1-40, 1988.
42. Peterson, V. M., Moore, E. E., Jones, T. N., *et al.* Total enteral nutrition versus total parenteral nutrition after major torso injury: Attenuation of hepatic protein reprioritization. *Surgery* 104:199-207, 1988.
43. Mochizuki, H., Trocki, O., Dominioni, L., *et al.* Mechanism of prevention of postburn hypermetabolism and catabolism by early enteral feeding. *Ann Surg* 200:297-310, 1984.
44. Dominioni, L., Trocki, O., Mochizuki, H., *et al.* Prevention of severe postburn hypermetabolism and catabolism by immediate intragastric feeding. *J Burn Care Rehabil* 5:106-112, 1984.
45. Jenkins, M., Gottschlich, M., Alexander, J. W., *et al.* Effect of immediate enteral feeding on the hypermetabolic response following severe burn injury. *JPEN* 13(Suppl 1):12S (Abstract), 1989.
46. Moore, E. E., and Jones, T. N. Benefits of immediate jejunostomy feeding after major abdominal trauma: A prospective, randomized study. *J Trauma* 26:874-880, 1986.
47. Pinilla, J. C., Oleniuk, F. H., Reed, D., *et al.* Does antacid prophylaxis prevent upper gastrointestinal bleeding in critically ill patients? *Crit Care Med* 13:646-650, 1985.
48. Cheadle, W. G., Vitale, G. C., Mackie, C. R., *et al.* Prophylactic postoperative nasogastric decompression. A prospective study of its requirement and the influence of cimetidine in 200 patients. *Ann Surg* 202:361-367, 1985.
49. DuMoulin, G. C., Paterson, D. G., Hedley-White, J., *et al.* Aspiration of gastric bacteria in antacid-treated patients: A frequent cause of postoperative colonisation of the airway. *Lancet* I:242-245, 1982.
50. Hillman, K. M., Riordan, T., O'Farrell, S. M., *et al.* Colonization of the gastric content in critically ill patients. *Crit Care Med* 10:444-448, 1982.
51. Kahn, R. J., Brimioulle, S., and Vincent, J. L. Influence of antacid treatment on the tracheal flora in mechanically ventilated patients. *Crit Care Med* 10:229 (Abstract), 1982.
52. Driks, M. R., Craven, D. E., Celli, B. R., *et al.* Nosocomial pneumonia in intubated patients randomized to sucralfate versus antacids and/or histamine type 2 blockers: The role of gastric colonization. *N Engl J Med* 317:1376-1382, 1987.
53. Goularte, T. A., Lichtenberg, D. A., and Craven, D. E. Gastric colonization in patients receiving antacids and mechanical ventilation: A mechanism for pharyngeal colonization. *Am J Infect Control* 14:88 (Abstract), 1986.
54. Garvey, B. M., McCambley, J. A., and Tuxen, D. V. Effects of gastric alkalinization on bacterial colonization in critically ill patients. *Crit Care Med* 17:211-216, 1989.
55. Kappstein, I., Vogel, W., Krieg, N., *et al.* The influence of exogenous and endogenous factors on the incidence of aspiration pneumonia. In: *Prevention of Stress Bleeding in Critically Ill Patients: A New Concept.* M. Tryba, Ed. Thieme, New York, 1988, pp. 105-122.

56. Tryba, M. Pulmonary complications during the prevention of stress bleeding with drugs. In: *Prevention of Stress Bleeding in Critically Ill Patients: A New Concept.* M. Tryba, Ed. Thieme, New York, 1988, pp. 128-135.

57. Tryba, M. Prevention of stress bleeding with ranitidine or pirenzepine and the risk of pneumonia. *J Clin Anesth* 1:12-20, 1988.

58. Craven, D. E., Kunchis, L. M., Kilinsky, V., *et al.* Risk factors for pneumonia and fatality in patients receiving continuous mechanical ventilation. *Am Rev Respir Dis* 133:792-796, 1986.

59. Atherton, S. T., and White, D. J. Stomach as source of bacteria colonising respiratory tract during artificial ventilation. *Lancet* II:968-969, 1978.

60. Johanson, W. G., Pierce, A. K., Sanford, J., *et al.* Nosocomial respiratory infections with gram negative bacilli: The significance of colonization of the respiratory tract. *Ann Intern Med* 77:701-706, 1972.

61. Tryba, M. The risk of acute stress bleeding and nosocomial pneumonia in ventilated ICU-patients: Sucralfate versus antacids. *Am J Med* 83(3B):117-124, 1987.

62. Cannon, L. A., Heiselman, D., Gardner, W., *et al.* Prophylaxis of upper gastrointestinal tract bleeding in mechanically ventilated patients: A randomized study comparing the efficacy of sucralfate, cimetidine, and antacids. *Arch Intern Med* 147:2101-2106, 1987.

63. Tryba, M., and Rether, J. Sucralfate versus antacids for the prevention of acute stress bleeding in risk patients receiving respiratory assistance. In: *Prevention of Stress Bleeding in Critically Ill Patients: A New Concept.* M. Tryba, Ed. Thieme, New York, 1988, pp. 42-49.

64. Laggner, A. N., Lenz, K., Stanek, G., *et al.* Bacterial colonization of the gastric juice of intensive care patients receiving stress ulcer prophylaxis: Sucralfate versus ranitidine. In: *Prevention of Stress Bleeding in Critically Ill Patients: A New Concept.* M. Tryba, Ed. Thieme, New York, 1988, pp. 123-127.

65. Silk, D. B. A., Fairclough, P. D., Clark, M. L., *et al.* Use of a peptide rather than free amino acid nitrogen source in chemically defined "elemental" diets. *JPEN* 4:548-553, 1980.

66. Brinson, R. R. Enteral nutrition in the critically ill patient: The role of hypoalbuminemia. In: *The Gastrointestinal Response to Injury, Starvation, and Enteral Nutrition.* 8th Ross Conference on Medical Research, Ross Laboratories, Columbus, Ohio, 1988, pp. 59-61.

67. Keohane, D. P., Grimble, G. K., Brown, B., *et al.* Influence of protein composition and hydrolysis method on intestinal absorption in man. *Gut* 26:907-913, 1985.

68. McArdle, A. H., and Bounous, G. Enteroprotection by elemental diets: Role of enteral feeding as prophylaxis against radiation injury. In: *The Gastrointestinal Response to Injury, Starvation, and Enteral Nutrition.* 8th Ross Conference on Medical Research, Ross Laboratories, Columbus, Ohio, 1988, pp. 68-70.

69. Hugon, J., and Bounous, G. Elemental diet in the management of the intestinal lesions produced by radiation in the mouse. *Can J Surg* 15:18-26, 1972.

70. Beer, W. H., Fan, A., and Halsted, C. H. Clinical and nutritional implication of radiation enteritis. *Am J Clin Nutr* 41:85-91, 1985.

71. Meredith, J. W., Ditesheim, J. A., and Zaloga, G. P. Visceral protein synthesis is greater with peptide-diet versus intact-protein diet in trauma patients. *J Trauma*, 29:1033 (Abstract), 1989.

72. Brinson, R. R., and Pitts, W. M. Enteral nutrition in the critically ill patient: Role of hypoalbuminemia. *Crit Care Med* 17:367-370, 1989.

73. Brinson, R. R., and Kolts, B. E. Diarrhea associated with severe hypoalbuminemia: A comparison of a peptide-based chemically defined diet and a standard enteral alimentation. *Crit Care Med* 16:130-136, 1988.

74. Poullain, M. G., Broyart, J. P., Roger, L., *et al.* Effect of whey proteins and their constitutive peptides or amino acids mixture on growth steatorrhea and nitrogen balance after acute starvation in the rat. *JPEN* 11:23S (Abstract), 1987.

75. Rerat, A., Nunes, C. S., Mendy, F., *et al.* Amino acid absorption and production of pancreatic hormones in non-anaesthetized pigs after duodenal infusions of a milk enzymic hydrolysate or of free amino acids. *Br J Nutr* 60:121-136, 1988.

76. Attebery, H. R., Sutter, V. L., and Finegold, S. M. Effect of a partially chemically defined diet on normal human fecal flora. *Am J Clin Nutr* 25:1391-1398, 1972.
77. Wilkins, T. D., and Long, W. R. Changes in the flora of the cecal mucosa of mice fed a chemically defined diet. *Bacteriol Proc* 71:113 (Abstract), 1971.
78. Bounous, G., LeBel, E., Schuster, J., et al. Dietary protection during radiation therapy. *Strahlenther Onkol* 149:476-483, 1975.

Role of Hematopoietic Growth Factors in Radiation Victims

RhGM-CSF Following the Goiânia Accident

Anna Butturini and Robert Peter Gale

Introduction

Total-body exposure to > 1 Gy of ionizing radiation at dose rates > 1 cGy per minute suppresses hematopoiesis in humans. Severity of bone marrow inhibition, duration of decreased blood cell levels, and likelihood of spontaneous recovery are dose dependent in the range of 1-10 Gy. Although experimental and clinical data suggest that some hematopoietic stem cells survive doses of radiation $\geq$ 10 Gy, hematopoietic recovery is unlikely at higher doses because of toxicity to nonhematopoietic organs or because supportive measures are unable to prolong survival long enough for recovery.[1-3]

Survival in persons receiving 1-9 Gy total-body radiation reflects a balance between the rate of hematologic recovery and the risk of death from infections or hemorrhage. Therapy is directed at preventing and treating infections by decreasing environmental and endogenous pathogens through the use of protected environments and antibiotics. Infections should be treated promptly. Granulocyte transfusions are ineffective.[4] Hemorrhage can be prevented by transfusing platelets.

A second strategy for treating radiation-related bone marrow failure is to replace the damaged hematopoietic system by an allogeneic or syngeneic bone marrow transplant. This approach was used in previous radiation accidents[5-7] and is discussed elsewhere in this volume.

A third approach to radiation-related hematopoietic suppression is to use hematopoietic growth factors to accelerate autologous bone marrow recovery. Several of these factors that act on different hematopoietic precursor cells have been cloned molecularly. Currently, recombinant human granulocyte-

A. BUTTURINI, Department of Pediatrics, Division of Hematology and Oncology, University of Parma, Parma 43100, Italy; R. P. GALE, Department of Medicine, Division of Hematology-Oncology, School of Medicine, University of California, Los Angeles, California 90024-1678.

Treatment of Radiation Injuries, Edited by
D. Browne *et al.,* Plenum Press, New York, 1990

macrophage colony-stimulating factor (rhGM-CSF), erythropoietin, granulocyte colony-stimulating factor (G-CSF), interleukin-3 (IL-3), and megakaryocyte colony-stimulating factor are available for experimental and clinical studies. The efficacy of these growth factors in persons with bone marrow failure is being studied.[8-9]

We used rhGM-CSF to stimulate myeloid recovery in persons who developed granulocytopenia after exposure to cesium-137 in a radiation accident in Goiânia, Brazil.[10] In this chapter, we review the results and discuss the use of hematopoietic growth factors in this setting.

Use of GM-CSF After the Goiânia Accident

In 1987, 10 persons living in Goiânia Brazil, developed granulocytopenia after external and internal exposure to cesium-137 (see table 1); details are reported elsewhere.[10] The time of exposure to cesium-137 was prolonged (up to 14 days), resulting in estimated total-body doses of 2.5-7 Gy. Granulocytopenia (neutrophils $< 1 \times 10^9$/L) developed 11-40 days after initial exposure. Seven persons also had thrombocytopenia and anemia requiring transfusions.

RhGM-CSF (activity 10^7 U/mg, Immunex Corporation, Seattle, WA, and Behringwerke AG, Marburg, FRG) became available 35 days after the accident. Treatment was immediately begun in eight persons (patients 3 through 10)

Table 1. Characteristics of 10 Patients with Responses to rhGM-CSF Treatment After the Goiânia Accident

Patient number	Sex	Age	Estimated dose (Gy)	Days to onset of neutropenia[1]	Days of neutropenia[1] before rhGM-CSF	Neutrophils ($\times 10^9$/L) Pretreatment	Peak	Outcome
1	M	22	6.2	20	(2)	(2)	(2)	Survival
2	M	36	7.1	12	(2)	(2)	(2)	Survival
3	F	37	6.0	11	10	0	0.6	Death (hemorrhage)
4	F	6	6.0	19	4	0	NE	Death (hemorrhage)
5	M	22	4.0	18	3	0.2	0.6	Death (pneumonia)
6	M	18	5.3	24	4	0.1	23.1	Death (pneumonia)
7	F	57	4.3	16	5	0.1	21.5	Survival
8	M	19	2.5	27	5	0	19.7	Survival
9	M	42	4.4	40	1	0.7	9.9	Survival
10	M	21	3.0	33	4	0.5	7.3	Survival

NE, not evaluable.
[1]Neutrophil counts were $< 1 \times 10^9$/L.
[2]Patients 1 and 2 were not considered for rhGM-CSF therapy.

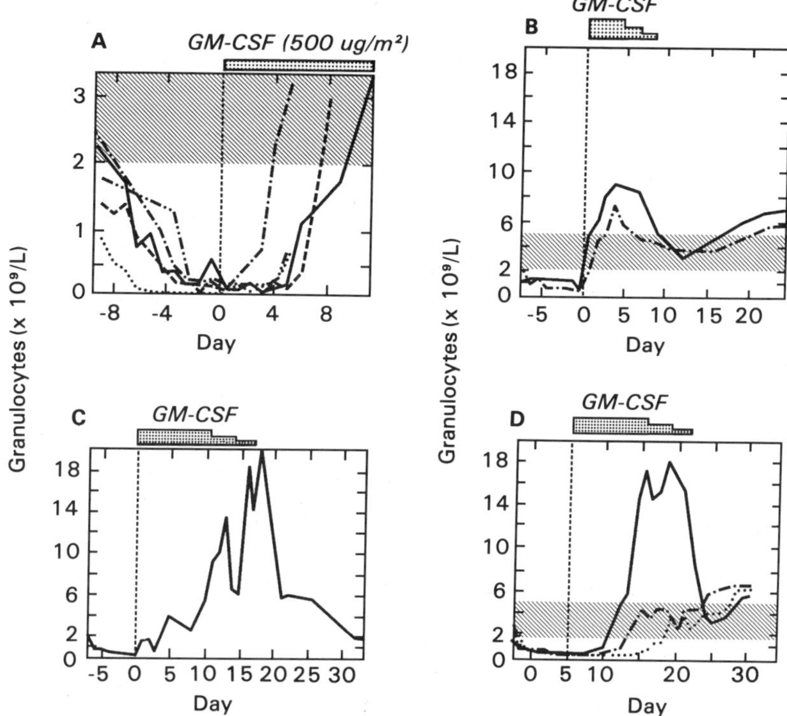

Figure 1. Responses to rHuGM-CSF [rhGM-CSF]. Curves adjusted such that day 0 is start of therapy:
(A) · · · = patient 3; –··– = patient 5; - - - = patient 6;   - · - = patient 7; —— = patient 8.
(B) —— = patient 9; - · - = patient 10. Initial dose of rHuGM-CSF [rhGM-CSF] 500 μg/m² per day.
(C) Patient 8. Initial dose 500 μg/m² per day.
(D) Granulocyte recovery in patients 1 (- · -) and 2 (· · ·) (no rHuGM-CSF [rhGM-CSF]), and in patient 8 (——) (initial dose of rHuGM-CSF [rhGM-CSF] 500 μg/m² per day). Curves adjusted to granulocytes < 0.5 x 10⁹/L on day 0.
(Reprinted with permission by *Lancet*.)

without any sign of spontaneous hematologic recovery at that time. Dosage of rhGM-CSF was 500 μg/m²/day in 24-hour infusions until neutrophils were > 2 x 10⁹/L for 3 consecutive days. Doses were reduced in 50-percent decrements when the neutrophil level was sustained.

In six persons (patients 3 through 8), rhGM-CSF treatment was initiated 4-11 days after the onset of severe granulocytopenia (neutrophils < 0.5 x 10⁹/L). All were colonized by resistant *Klebsiella* species; two had bacterial sepsis. Treatment of patients 9 and 10 began when neutrophils were 0.7 x 10⁹/L and 0.5 x 10⁹/L, respectively.

Four of the eight patients died of gram-negative sepsis 6-9 days after beginning treatment. Patient 4 could not be evaluated for the effect of GM-CSF because she died within hours of beginning GM-CSF therapy without signs of recovery. All had high fevers and positive cultures for multiantibiotic-resistant *Klebsiella*. The cause of death in two subjects was diffuse internal hemorrhage, and the other two died of rapidly evolving pneumonia and shock unresponsive to antibiotics and vasopressors.

In seven of the eight subjects, neutrophils reached $> 0.5 \times 10^9/L$ 1-5 days after rhGM-CSF was initiated (figure 1). Their platelet and red cell recovery seemed unaffected.

In the four survivors (patients 7 through 10), duration of rhGM-CSF treatment was 8-14 days. One of the four developed high fever, pneumonia, and hypotension after 10 days of treatment; neutrophils were $9.1 \times 10^9/L$. A gram-negative organism was isolated from blood culture, and the patient recovered after receiving antibiotics. The three other subjects recovered uneventfully.

After treatment was discontinued, the survivors' neutrophil levels returned to normal within 3-5 days (see figure 1). During the 18-month follow-up period, neutrophils remained normal in three persons; the fourth (patient 7) developed a mild decrease in neutrophils $(1 \text{ to } 2 \times 10^9/L)$, which began 1 month after discontinuing rhGM-CSF (A. R. Oliveira, personal communication).

Discussion

Three concepts underlie the use of hematopoietic growth factors after radiation accidents. The first relates to the persistence of hematopoietic progenitors. Previous data suggest that persons receiving estimated doses of total-body radiation > 9 Gy in accidents can recover autologous hematopoiesis.[5,6] This effect may be related to the radioresistance of some stem cells, to repair of sublethal radiation damage, or possibly to nonuniform radiation exposure or dose fractionation.

The second concept relates to the efficacy of treatment. Several clinical and preclinical studies indicate that rhGM-CSF, rhG-CSF, and IL-3 enhance hematologic recovery in subjects receiving cytotoxic chemotherapy or bone marrow transplants.[11-15] In the Goiânia accident, persons treated with rhGM-CSF showed a different rate and pattern of neutrophil recovery compared to untreated persons (figure 1). This observation and the rapid decline in neutrophils when treatment was discontinued suggest that rhGM-CSF affected myeloid recovery. This suggestion is consistent with data in irradiated animals (T. J. MacVittie, this volume). Furthermore, GM-CSF treatment might prevent prolonged granulocytopenia in persons treated immediately when neutrophils are $< 1 \times 10^9/L$.

The third concept relates to safety. Early side effects of rhGM-CSF treatment are fever and phlebitis. Neutrophil accumulation at sites of prior infection, pulmonary infiltrates and edema, capillary leak syndrome, and shock are reported, especially after higher doses (> 30 μg/kg/day) in persons treated with rhGM-CSF. Side effects of rhG-CSF seem milder.[11-17]

After the Goiânia accident, three of the subjects who were receiving rhGM-CSF developed respiratory failure and shock. All had gram-negative bacteremia. Although respiratory failure was ascribed to infection, we cannot exclude an effect of rhGM-CSF. It is interesting that the person who developed gram-negative sepsis when neutrophils were > 9 x 10^9/L survived. One other subject had mild fever during the rhGM-CSF infusion. Potential long-term consequences of rhGM-CSF treatment relate to a possible alteration in the balance between self-renewal and differentiation of stem cells. Also, stem cells driven to proliferate may be more sensitive to radiation, particularly if exposure continues. This sensitivity could be important in persons with internal radiation contamination. Increased damage also might occur if proliferating cells have less opportunity to repair radiation-induced abnormalities. One or more of these effects might result in depletion of the stem-cell pool and, consequently, in late failure of hematopoiesis. No data to support this hypothesis are currently available from persons receiving rhG-CSF and rhGM-CSF during chemotherapy or following radiation. In irradiated dogs, however, treatment with IL-3 causes early increases in granulocytes, followed by delayed or absent bone marrow recovery (T. J. MacVittie, personal communication). One of four persons treated with rhGM-CSF who survived the Goiânia accident developed mild granulocytopenia 18 months after discontinuing rhGM-CSF; bone marrow cellularity was normal. Antibodies to rhGM-CSF and studies of clonogenic myeloid precursor cells have not been investigated yet.

It is not known which growth factors, either alone or in combination, should be used in radiation accidents, nor are the optimal timing and schedule of administration clear. Data for irradiated animals clearly demonstrate that rhGM-CSF and rhG-CSF accelerate granulocyte recovery; erythropoiesis and thrombopoiesis are usually unaffected. Combinations with other growth factors, such as IL-1 and IL-3, are probably active on more primitive stem cells; human data are lacking.

Data from the Goiânia accident suggest that early treatment with rhGM-CSF reduces granulocytopenia with minimal adverse effects. It also appears that treatment with rhGM-CSF may have increased survival. Treatment seemed more effective when given early.

References

1. United Nations Scientific Committee on Atomic Radiation. *Sources, Effects and Risks of Ionizing Radiation.* 1988 Report to the General Assembly with Annexes. United Nations, NY, 1988.

2. Gale, R. P. Immediate medical consequences of nuclear accidents: Lessons from Chernobyl. *JAMA* 258:625-628, 1987.
3. Barabanova, A. B., Baranov, A. E., Guskova, A. K., *et al. Acute Radiation Effects in Man.* National Committee on Radiation Protection, Moscow, 1986.
4. Winston, D. J., Ho, W. G., Gale, R. P., *et al.* Therapeutic granulocyte transfusions for documented infections: A controlled trial of ninety-five infectious granulocytopenic episodes. *Ann Intern Med* 97:509-515, 1982.
5. Jammet, H., Mathe, G., Pendic, B., *et al.* Study of six cases of accidental acute total-body irradiation. *Rev Fr Etud Clin Biol* 4:210-225, 1959.
6. Gale, R. P., and Reisner, Y. The role of bone marrow transplants after nuclear accidents. *Lancet* I:923-925, 1988.
7. Baranov, A., Gale, R. P., Guskova, A. K., *et al.* Bone marrow transplantation after the Chernobyl nuclear accident. *N Engl J Med* 321:205-212, 1989.
8. Dexter, M. Growth factors: From the laboratory to the clinic. *Nature* 321:198, 1986.
9. Nienhuis, A. W. Hematopoietic growth factors. *N Engl J Med* 318:916-918, 1988.
10. Butturini, A., De Souza, P. C., Gale, R. P., *et al.* Use of recombinant granulocyte-macrophage colony-stimulating factor in the Brazil radiation accident. *Lancet* II:471-475, 1988.
11. Brandt, S. J., Peters, W. P., Atwater, S. K., *et al.* Effect of recombinant human granulocyte-macrophage colony-stimulating factor on hematopoietic reconstitution after high dose chemotherapy and bone marrow transplantation. *N Engl J Med* 318:869-876, 1988.
12. Gabrilove, J. L., Jakubowski, A., Scher, H., *et al.* Effect of granulocyte colony-stimulating factor on neutropenia and associated morbidity due to chemotherapy for transitional-cell carcinoma of the urothelium. *N Engl J Med* 318:1414-1422, 1988.
13. Vadhan-Raj, S., Keating, M., LeMaistre, A., *et al.* Effects of recombinant human granulocyte-macrophage colony-stimulating factor in patients with myelodysplastic syndromes. *N Engl J Med* 317:1545-1552, 1987.
14. Bronchud, M. H., Scarffe, J. H., Thatcher, N., *et al.* Phase I/II study of recombinant human granulocyte colony-stimulating factor in patients receiving intensive chemotherapy for small cell lung cancer. *Br J Cancer* 56:809-813, 1987.
15. Morstyn, G., Campbell, L., Sousa, L. M., *et al.* Effect of granulocyte colony-stimulating factor on neutropenia induced by cytotoxic chemotherapy. *Lancet* I:667-672, 1988.
16. Champlin, R. E., Nimer, S. D., Ireland, P., *et al.* Treatment of refractory aplastic anemia with recombinant granulocyte-macrophage colony-stimulating factor. *Blood* 73:694-699, 1989.
17. Steward, W. P., Scarffe, J. H., Austin, K., *et al.* Recombinant human granulocyte-macrophage colony-stimulating factor (rhGM-CSF) given as a daily short infusion: A phase I dose-toxicity study. *Br J Cancer* 59:142-145, 1989.

Infectious Complications

Roundtable Discussion
(Questions and discussions were summarized by the book editors.)

Question:

When should broad-spectrum versus single-agent antibiotic therapy be used?

Discussion:

Controversy exists as to whether single-agent therapy or combination therapy is the best approach for the treatment of infection in the immunocompromised, febrile, neutropenic host. Another controversy is whether coverage with vancomycin should be added for *Staphylococcus epidermidis* or other gram-positive organisms. Should we use single antibiotics, such as cephalosporins (ceftazidine) and imipenem with or without vancomycin, or should we use dual or triple antibiotic combinations of aminoglycosides with extended spectrum penicillin and/or cephalosporins?

The current consensus is that physicians should use the therapies with which they are most familiar in the particular clinical setting. If the physician is more comfortable using single-agent therapy, and the patient responds to it, then agents such as imipenem or ceftazidine would be adequate, although, in each setting, resistance may develop to any of these agents. For neutropenia, the current trend in the particular hospital setting should be considered, because some patients may not respond to treatment and may deteriorate rather rapidly. In the future, other agents, such as the quinolones (currently being studied), may be used to treat the immunocompromised host.

Question:

What are the recommendations for new modalities for reducing infections or infectious portals of entry, specifically, blocking the effects with magnetic and electric field gradients, heparin-bonding catheters, or epithelial growth factors? Are there any other ways to improve wound healing by preventing bacterial adhesion to inert surfaces?

Discussion:

The standard treatment is to rotate catheters frequently; intravenous lines should be removed every 3 days, and peripheral lines and central lines should be replaced every 5-6 days. There are two new systems available that will probably be better for peripheral access. Catheters with antibiotic-impregnated cuffs that fit at the site of entry are available now. These cuffs decrease the colonization of the catheter, which indicates that most of the bacteria come from the skin. Studies have shown that if peripheral lines are left in more than 3 days, infection rates go up tremendously. The data on these new catheters show that they can be left in 5-6 days.

Question:

When is the best time to start and finish antibiotic therapy? Is there any advantage in starting empiric or prophylactic therapy in a severely neutropenic patient before the onset of fever?

Discussion:

Initiate the antibiotic therapy coverage when the fever reaches 37°C and neutropenia is present also. Neutropenia alone does not require antibiotic treatment. Data from immunocompromised and bone marrow transplant patients indicate that in all situations it is best to wait until fever occurs with neutropenia and not to give intravenous antibiotics prophylactically. Treat these patients like any other immunocompromised patients when discontinuing therapy. When the white blood cell count and the underlying infection are under control, then discontinue empiric antibiotics.

Continue to treat the patient as long as the fever is present, especially if it is associated with neutropenia, and even if it takes 2-3 weeks to bring the fever down and if the addition of antifungal agents is necessary. It is important to continue treatment as long as necessary. Routinely, use prophylactic antibiotics before surgery to prevent local or systemic infections. Several studies have shown that some antibiotics prevent dissemination of infection if used correctly, but the problem might be more difficult in the irradiated patient because of the suppression of the gut flora and problems with secondary infections. There is no set answer; the best clinical judgment of the physician should be used. If palliative surgery must be performed in an area heavily contaminated with bacteria, then the physician may be forced to use antibiotics. However, it is recommended that such usage be restricted to a short period of time, especially if the operation is performed during the first 48 hours after radiation exposure, while some immune functions still remain.

Question:

What is the recommended method of controlling cytomegalovirus (CMV) infections?

Discussion:

The problems of the neutropenic radiation victim are similar to those of the patient undergoing bone marrow transplantation. Bone marrow transplantation patients also receive a high radiation exposure if a total-body irradiation regimen is used. Several studies have shown that total-body irradiation induces as much as 70-80 percent reactivation of oral mucocutaneous or genital herpes simplex virus, often by the seventh day after exposure. A series of studies done on the marrow transplant population in antibody-positive patients showed that oral acyclovir markedly reduces or virtually eliminates the development of mucocutaneous herpes simplex viral infections. Thus, oral acyclovir is the standard treatment for antibody-positive, neutropenic, irradiated patients for prevention of herpes simplex. If oral acyclovir is given prophylactically, and if severe mucocitis develops unrelated to herpes, then intravenous acyclovir can be given. Gancyclovir for CMV infections is being clinically tested under restricted Food and Drug Administration (FDA) protocols. Currently, gancyclovir provides only temporary relief from retinitis; when the drug is stopped, retinitis recurs.

In a series of patients with CMV pneumonitis, which was fatal a few years ago, treatment with gancyclovir and high-dose gamma globulin rescued 70 percent of patients. Gancyclovir was approved by the FDA for limited protocols of compassionate use.

Question:

Did the patients from Goiânia, Brazil, with bone marrow depression become refractory to platelet transfusion?

Discussion:

No. There were only three patients requiring platelet transfusions, and transfusions were given for less than 1 month. The highest number of transfusions was about eight—too few to cause the patient to become refractory to platelet transfusion.

Question:

Are there any current issues of importance regarding the use of parenteral versus enteral nutrition in irradiated patients? Would decisions for parenteral or enteral nutrition be different for irradiated patients, compared with patients who are immunosuppressed for other reasons?

Discussion:

The absorption of nutrients by the gut could be different in the irradiated individual. Combined injury with or without sepsis may affect nutrient absorption in the irradiated patient and help to determine whether parenteral or enteral nutrition would be advisable. With regard to differences in absorption by the irradiated intestine, there is evidence that inhibition of amino acid transport is not due to inhibition of cellular sodium potassium ATPase. The cells remaining on the villi are quite capable of absorbing amino acids, and animal studies indicate that isolated cells have increased glucose transport after irradiation. Therefore, the cells on the villi are apparently quite capable of absorbing both glucose and amino acids, and it is only when the cells are no longer present that inhibition develops.

A substance in the circulation of critically ill patients inhibits sodium and potassium transport. A so-called endogenous digoxinlike substance that may affect mainly red cells has been isolated. There is evidence that, with radiation exposure alone, transport processes are intact for epithelial cells in the intestine. No data exist on cell transport processes for patients with combined injury.

Depending on the dose and time of irradiation, it may not be wise to start oral feeding of irradiated individuals immediately. Many of these individuals may suffer from suppressed gastric emptying, resulting in stasis of oral intake. The effect of supplemental diets and oral rehydration is being reviewed in consideration of the suppressed gastric emptying. The dose of radiation and its effect on gastric emptying should influence the decision of whether to administer food or various drugs orally.

Studies using radio-contrast dye on patients with poor gastric emptying show that food moves through the stomach fairly well—it may be slowed but it does go through. If oral feedings must be continued, they should be given in a controlled, long-term manner. Gastric emptying becomes a problem when too much food is given too fast or a bolus-type feeding is given.

Question:

What is the role of enteral nutrition in patients with a leaky gut due to the gastrointestinal syndrome after radiation exposure?

Discussion:

Little is known about this problem. The gut is primarily a luminally fed organ; if you do not feed the gut, the protein and villous structures will break down, and atrophy will occur. Recent clinical trials have tested supplemental intravenous glutamine with total parenteral nutrition. Animal studies show that this treatment allows the gut to grow back more quickly, preventing atrophy. However, glutamine is not stable in solution, and there may be a dose curve— too much glutamine may damage the mucosa. It is recommended that total parenteral nutrition supplemented with glutamine be used in minimal amounts to promote regrowth of the gut. More rapid feeding can be attempted when regeneration starts.

Question:

What is the most appropriate initial field treatment of irradiated casualties with respect to management of infection and nutrition in gut decontamination?

Discussion:

In the field, treatment protocols may not be ideal. Realistically, try to avoid as much contamination or ingestion of virulent organisms as possible. After triage of irradiated patients, try to minimize absorption of organisms by reducing the intake of food items that may contain bacteria, such as fresh fruits and vegetables. Use any available canned food and try to acidify the water or use iodine pills. Try to reduce the number of organisms in the gut with antibiotics that can be administered in the field, such as quinolones in pill form, which have a long shelf life. Quinolones are selective to aerobes in the gut, are absorbed systematically, and maintain a systemic level that can be therapeutic. Of course, resistance to quinolones can occur.

Question:

Are there any preclinical data supporting the use of immunomodulators in the treatment of radiation injury?

Discussion:

In a study using the canine model, we established gram-negative peritonitis by implanting bacteria in a fibrin clot intraperitoneally after a small laparotomy. Two models of sepsis were examined: (1) cardiac and pulmonary aspects of septic shock, and (2) multiple organ system failure. The only effective therapeutic protocol that increased mean survival time, as well as survival, involved the immediate use of fluids, such as Ringer's lactate, and a third-generation cephalosporin antibiotic; the immunomodulator glucan had no positive effect on survival when administered therapeutically. Work with monoclonal antibodies to endotoxin lipopolysaccharide (anti-J5) has been done, but the data are equivocal; there is no increase in survival whatsoever. Another modulator, lipid X, was tried, and it was also ineffective. However, this was a difficult study to evaluate because bacteria were implanted directly into the peritoneal cavity of the animal. Better results would be expected if the animals were pretreated with glucan.

The timing of administration of immunomodulators in immunocompromised patients is important. Experience with the application of antibiotics and immunomodulators in mouse models can, perhaps, be extrapolated to the human situation, taking into consideration the problems posed by peak efficacy time of some of these agents.

The efficacy of glucan, whether given before or after irradiation, depends greatly on the radiation dose as well as the time of administration. At a midlethal radiation dose ($\leq LD_{50/30}$), preirradiation or postirradiation therapy can be effective, even if it is administered as much as 1-2 weeks before or after irradiation. However, at higher radiation doses, where very few bone marrow stem cells would be expected to survive, treatment can be delayed for a maximum of 24 hours after irradiation and still achieve good results. Actually, in these circumstances, the best effect is achieved when glucan is given 1-3 hours after irradiation.

Immunomodulator therapy with glucan appears to enhance survival through at least two mechanisms: (1) activation of radioresistant macrophage populations, which can play a role in the control of postirradiation infection, and (2) stimulation of hematopoietic regeneration. The immunomodulator trehalose dimycolate (TDM) administered to normal or sublethally irradiated mice has also been demonstrated to stimulate macrophage function, based on the ability to engulf and kill bacteria.

If mice are challenged with a dose of *Klebsiella pneumoniae* 4 days after sublethal irradiation, less than 100 organisms will kill them by day 8. If bacterial infection develops after irradiation, as much time as possible is needed for TDM to be effective in the animal. This immunomodulator was also studied in mice in combination with cephalosporin treatment. Animals were treated with TDM immediately after irradiation, then challenged with bacteria on the fourth day after irradiation. Cephalosporin treatment started on the day after bacterial challenge. All the animals were rescued by this treatment, whereas 80 percent survived with cephalosporin treatment only. TDM was most effective when given 1 hour after irradiation, and the efficacy decreased when the time was extended.

Combined Injury
Complications

The Status of Combined Injuries

Erwin F. Hirsch

Introduction

The association of blunt-penetrating trauma, thermal burns, and radiation injury has been witnessed only once—after the detonation of atomic bombs over Hiroshima and Nagasaki in 1945. In the years that followed, many lessons were learned from the survivors, but little documentation of the medical effects of these combined injuries is available.

During the subsequent four decades, a variety of accidents involving ionizing radiation were documented; most of the accidents occurred shortly after World War II and were related to the processing of nuclear weapons, medical mishaps, or industrial accidents due largely to the mismanagement of radioisotopes. Soft-tissue injuries occurred occasionally as a consequence of radiation injury, but combined injuries as seen in Japan were never again documented.[1,2]

On April 26, 1986, however, a major malfunction occurred in a nuclear reactor in Chernobyl, U.S.S.R. Evacuation of 135,000 persons was required; of the 237 persons admitted with signs and symptoms of acute radiation syndrome, 27 had sustained either thermal burns or radiation burns (table 1). Thirty-one patients died, and the combination of dermal pathology and radiation injury carried a poor prognosis.

In October 1987, the mishandling of a radiation therapy unit in Goiânia, Brazil, was responsible for the contamination of 244 patients with cesium-137. Although no simultaneous injuries occurred, the clinical and laboratory observations that were made are useful for understanding the pathophysiology of combined injuries.

E. F. HIRSCH, Department of Surgery, Boston University Medical Center, Boston, Massachusetts 02118, and Department of Surgery, Uniformed Services University of the Health Sciences, Bethesda, Maryland 20814.

Treatment of Radiation Injuries, Edited by
D. Browne *et al.*, Plenum Press, New York, 1990

Table 1. Chernobyl Patient Classification

Radiation injury	Dose (Gy)	Number of patients		
		Total	Deaths[1]	Burns
Slight	1-2	140	0	0
Moderate	2-4	55	1	0
Severe	4-6	21	7	6
Extremely severe	6-10	21	20	20[2]

[1]In addition, one person was unaccounted for, and one patient died within 4 hours of the accident.
[2]Body surface area equals 40-90 percent.

Background

The synergistic effects of total-body irradiation and trauma and/or burns have been established for about 25 years. Sheep exposed to 4 Gy total-body irradiation and thereafter subjected to barotrauma suffered increased mortality from 25 percent to 50 percent. Messerschmidt *et al.* established that mortality increased from 26 percent to 90 percent when cutaneous wounds followed total-body irradiation.[3-5]

Ledney *et al.*[6] further established that the timing of the injury and exposure to radiation altered outcome and that survival improved if the trauma injury preceded radiation injury. The synergistic effects of total-body irradiation and thermal injury were documented by several investigators.[7-9] Messerschmidt established that mortality from both total-body irradiation and thermal injury increased from 10 percent singly to 90 percent combined. Alpen and Sheline[10] described the significant increase in mortality when 1 Gy, 2.5 Gy, and 5 Gy of total-body irradiation were superimposed on an LD_{50} burn wound model; the mortalities increased to 65 percent, 90 percent, and 100 percent, respectively.

Although increased lethality has been observed in a number of animal models, until recently no major studies had been undertaken to establish the immunologic, metabolic, and hematopoietic changes associated with combined injuries. Furthermore, except for some of Messerschmidt's work related to the response of wound closure after combined injuries, no major studies of the surgical management of combined injuries have been carried out.

Pathophysiology of Combined Injuries

Similarities between ionizing radiation injuries and trauma injuries could explain the synergistic effects observed in experimental models.

Even in sublethal doses, ionizing radiation compromises the hematopoietic and gastrointestinal (GI) systems. Depending on the dose, the reproductive capabilities of the hematopoietic stem cells are strongly inhibited, and peripheral cellular forms are consequently depleted. Lymphocytes are significantly decreased in humans after 24 hours, granulocytes in several days, and platelets in 10-14 days. Anemia occurs early as a result of hemorrhage and later as a result of bone marrow suppression. The magnitude of exposure can be estimated retrospectively in patients or animals by the rate of depletion of the respective cells and their eventual recovery. The critical manifestation of the hematopoietic phase of the acute radiation syndrome can be characterized by pancytopenia, clinical coagulopathies, and eventual systemic sepsis. As sensitive as the bone marrow, but not so well understood, are the responses of the GI system to total-body irradiation. Small-bowel epithelium is as sensitive as the bone marrow and plays an important role in the potential for survival after irradiation. Loss and decreased production of cells covering the villi are characteristic of exposure to relatively low doses of total-body irradiation. Disruption of the tight cell junctions of the intestinal mucosa was observed in animal models and may be responsible for the development of endogenous endotoxemia and bacteremia by allowing microorganisms access to the portal and lymphatic circulation. The clinical symptoms include diarrhea, vomiting, malabsorption, electrolyte imbalance, malnutrition, and sepsis.

Mortality after burns or serious musculoskeletal trauma follows a trimodal distribution. The first peak of deaths occurs immediately after the accident or in transit to the hospital. The second peak occurs during the first few hours of hospitalization; in most instances, these deaths are the result of inappropriate early assessment and delays in management. The successful early management of the significantly injured patient, however, does not diminish the risk for major septic complications, which may eventually jeopardize functional rehabilitation or cause death, usually from multisystem failure—the third peak. Although errors in management and nosocomial sepsis are sometimes partly responsible for septic complications, the physiological and anatomical magnitude of the injuries is associated with cellular, humoral, and immunologic changes and metabolic abnormalities that render the patients immunodeficient and susceptible to septic complications.

The goal in the management of these patients, therefore, is to minimize the stresses and to support or enhance the mechanisms that protect the host from septic complications.

Diagnostic and Therapeutic Management

Early evaluation and aggressive resuscitation of the trauma/burn patient are paramount after combined injuries. Airway management, oxygenation, ventilation, and resuscitation from hypovolemia need to be carried out expeditiously. Replacement of oxygen-carrying capacity by means of blood transfusions will require, however, that all blood be previously irradiated to prevent the transfusion of live white cells. This practice was standard during the management of the Chernobyl and Goiânia patients. The magnitude of the thermal or musculoskeletal injuries such casualties exhibit should be easily assessed by standard protocols. The magnitude of radiation injury, however, may be difficult or impossible to assess during the resuscitative phase of treatment. The decision for early management, therefore, should be based on observation of the patient's signs and symptoms. Simultaneous efforts should be made to record observations pertaining to the acute radiation syndrome and to obtain the biological samples that will establish the magnitude of the radiation injury.

The dynamics of the acute radiation syndrome are such that a successful outcome from surgical intervention may be possible only during a brief period of time after the injury. When surgical procedures are necessary, they should be performed no later than 3-4 days after the accident.

Catabolism, immunosuppression, and other changes that are characteristic of the host with an open wound are well known. Limited experience with animals in the field of combined injuries seems to indicate that wound closure significantly improves outcome. The closure of wounds after major trauma is usually not indicated or technically feasible. In those situations, the use of biological wound dressings may allow the host to respond in a way that minimizes mortality or morbidity.

References

1. Conklin, J. J., Walker, R., and Hirsch, E. F. Current concepts in the management of radiation injuries and associated trauma. *Surg Gynecol Obstet* 156:809-829, 1983.
2. Bowers, G. J. The combined injury syndrome. In: *Military Radiobiology.* J. J. Conklin and R. I. Walker, Eds. Academic Press, Orlando, 1987, pp. 191-217.
3. Messerschmidt, O. E. Strahlenbelastung und offene hautwunde. *Arch Klin Exp Dermatol* 227:329-335, 1966.
4. Stromberg, L. W. R., Woodward, K. T., Mahan, D. T., et al. Combined surgical and radiation injury. *Ann Surg* 167:18-22, 1968.
5. Drouet, J., Monpeyssin, M., Dubos, M., et al. *Etude des lesion combines associant irradiation et blessures experimentales. (Studies of combined injuries, the combination of irradiation and experimental burns.)* Centre de Recherches du Service de Sante des Armees, Clamart, France, 1982.
6. Ledney, G. D., Exum, E. D., and Sheehy, P. A. Survival enhanced by skin wound trauma in mice exposed to ^{60}Co radiation. *Experientia* 37:193-194, 1981.
7. Brooks, J. W., Evans, E. I., Ham, W. T., et al. The influence of external body radiation on mortality from thermal burns. *Ann Surg* 136:533-545, 1952.
8. Baker, D. G., and Valeriote, F. A. Effects of thermal burn and x-irradiation on early mortality. *Proc Soc Exp Biol Med* 121:1275-1279, 1966.
9. Messerschmidt, O., Birkenmayer, E., Bomes, H., et al. Radiation sickness combined with burns. IAEA-SM-119/34:173-179, 1970.
10. Alpen, F. L., and Sheline, G. E. The combined effects of thermal burns and whole body x-irradiation on survival time and mortality. *Ann Surg* 140:113-118, 1954.

Combined Radiation and Thermal Injury After Nuclear Attack

*William K. Becker, Teresa M. Buescher,
William G. Cioffi, William F. McManus,
and Basil A. Pruitt, Jr.*

Introduction

The explosion of nuclear weapons over the Japanese cities of Hiroshima and Nagasaki in 1945 dramatically changed the potential for thermally injured casualties as a result of warfare. Except for isolated radiation accidents over the ensuing years, little practical experience has been gained in the treatment of thermal injuries associated with radiation or nuclear warfare. In this chapter, we discuss the current status of burn care, review experimental animal data regarding combined injury of burns and radiation, and correlate the findings with the need to triage thermal injuries under the conditions of nuclear warfare.

Current Status of Burn Care

Thermal injuries are a common medical problem affecting more than 2 million individuals in the United States annually. Most of these injuries are minor and are treated on an outpatient basis. Between 60,000 and 70,000 patients per year are burned severely enough to require hospital treatment.[1] Major burn injury results in a systemic response characterized by an early period of shock with hypovolemia, gastrointestinal ileus, and oliguria. After adequate resuscitation, the burn patient converts to a hyperdynamic state characterized by increased cardiac output, diuresis, and peripheral catabolism.[2]

When nuclear weapons were used in 1945, there was little if any treatment available. Since that time, there have been a number of advances in the treatment of thermally injured patients, especially in the areas of fluid resuscitation, burn wound care, and surgical management of the burn wound. Investigators, including Harkins, Cope and Moore, Evans, and the group at the U.S. Army Institute of Surgical Research, defined plasma volume deficit

W. K. BECKER, T. M. BUESCHER, W. G. CIOFFI, W. F. McMANUS, and B. A. PRUITT, Jr., U.S. Army Institute of Surgical Research, Fort Sam Houston, Texas 78234-5012.

Treatment of Radiation Injuries, Edited by
D. Browne *et al.,* Plenum Press, New York, 1990

as the cause of early burn shock and developed resuscitation formulas that have essentially eliminated early death from burn shock and early acute renal failure.[3,4] As patients were successfully resuscitated from burn shock, sepsis became the major cause of death in thermally injured patients.[5] The introduction of penicillin and other systemic antibiotics changed the bacteriology of burn-wound infection from streptococcal organisms to other organisms, such as the *Staphylococcus and Pseudomonas aeruginosa*.[6] The development of topical chemotherapeutic agents, such as mafenide acetate and 0.5 percent silver nitrate, has resulted in a marked decrease in invasive burn wound infection by effectively controlling proliferation of bacteria.[7]

In addition to the development of effective resuscitation and topical chemotherapy, there have been other changes in the management of burn wounds. The trend recently has been to perform early excision of the burn wound, either tangentially or to the level of the investing fascia, and to close the wound early with the use of meshed autografts.[8] When donor sites are limited, the use of cadaver allograft or other biologic or synthetic skin substitutes has allowed the burn wound to be removed early and the wound to be covered temporarily, pending final closure with autograft.[9] During this time, there have also been changes in nutritional support, mechanical ventilation, invasive hemodynamic monitoring, and other aspects of general supportive care of critically ill patients.

Associated with these advances in burn care has been an improvement in patient survival, with the predominant improvement in young adults and middle-aged individuals with major burns. Figures from the early 1980's compared to those of the middle 1940's show an increase in LA_{50} (extent of burn that has been associated with death in 50 percent of patients) for young adults from 43 percent of the body surface to 59.6 percent (table 1). An improvement was also seen for individuals over 40 years of age. Figure 1 shows these changes in mortality, and illustrates the age, burn size, and percentage decrease in death rate at the U.S. Army Institute of Surgical Research from 1950-63 to 1980-86. In this three-dimensional representation, the major gains are noted in the young and middle-aged groups with burn size varying from 40 percent to 60 percent in the region of the LA_{50}.

Table 1. Survival Rate of Patients With Burns
From 1945-47 to 1980-84 (LA_{50})

Age of patient	Survival rate (percent)	
	1945-47	1980-84
15-40	43	59.6
Over 40	23	35.7

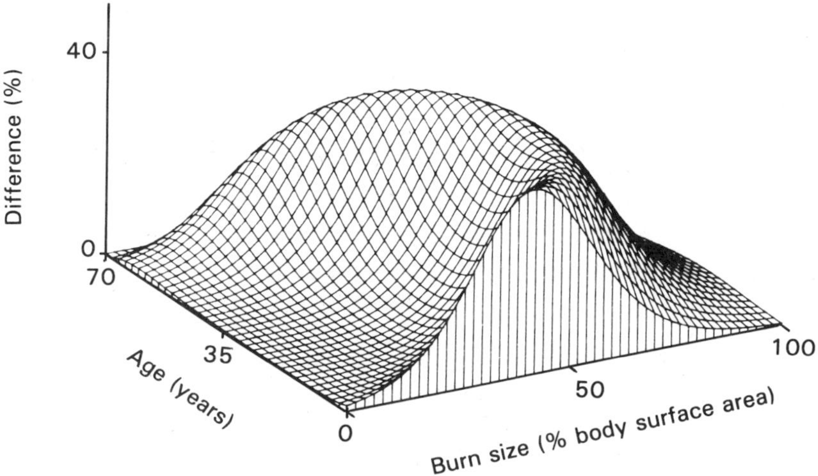

Figure 1. Decrease in number of deaths per 100 patients from 1950-1963 to 1980-1986 at the U.S. Army Institute of Surgical Research.

Logistics of Burn Care

In the United States, major burns (involving more than 20 percent of body surface area for adults) are best cared for at specialized burn centers. In 1987, 182 hospitals in the United States either had burn care units or specialized burn care programs. There were about 1,800 dedicated burn care beds. In 1985, of the approximately 70,000 patients requiring hospitalization for burns, 25-30 percent (about 21,000) were admitted to burn care facilities. Patients with major burns generally require 1 day of hospitalization for each percentage of the body surface area with second- or third-degree thermal injury. While in the intensive care unit, patients with thermal injuries require approximately 28 hours of nursing care per day, in addition to specialized care from respiratory therapists, occupational and physical therapists, dieticians, and pharmacists. Because patients require up to 9 percent of the blood volume for each 1 percent of the body surface area excised by the tangential technique, major burns can strain blood-banking services. It is clear from these statistics that only a limited number of patients can receive the quality and quantity of care required to achieve the survival rates previously described. However, most patients with minor thermal injuries do well with simple outpatient care, and do not require a substantial investment of resources.

Combined Injuries

The airburst detonation of a nuclear weapon over a population center will result in many thermal injuries. In addition to the thermal injuries, a significant number of survivors will also suffer some degree of radiation injury, either immediately or over the ensuing several weeks as a result of fallout. At Hiroshima and Nagasaki, from one-fourth to one-half of the survivors had some degree of thermal injury.[10]   Most of these injuries resulted from the flash of radiant heat from the detonation of the bomb. A small number resulted from flame burns caused by secondary fires. Only a small area of the body surface (up to 10 percent) was involved in most patients, because clothing or other objects in the path of the radiation provided significant protection. Because of the small size of the nuclear devices used in Hiroshima and Nagasaki, it is difficult to extrapolate these data to the larger weapons stored in military arsenals today. These larger devices are more likely to cause major fires, so-called superfires, when detonated over large population centers.[11]   Thus, the possibility exists for a significant increase in the number and size of burns resulting from direct flame, and burns often will be complicated by inhalation injury.[12]

The expected mortality from thermal injuries complicated by radiation injury in humans is unknown. In major burns, mortality rates similar to those described earlier could be expected if comprehensive care were available to the injured. If comprehensive care were unavailable, as is likely after a nuclear attack, mortality rates approaching 100 percent for patients with thermal injuries involving more than 30 percent of the body surface area could be expected. In all likelihood, individuals with burns on less than 20 percent of the body surface area would survive, although they would not receive specific treatment for a period of time.[13]   Many who have only partial thickness burns or minor full-thickness burns involving less than 10 percent of the body surface area could be expected to survive even without treatment. As the area involved with full-thickness injury exceeds 10 percent, increased mortality can be expected if treatment is unavailable. Mortality depends on the age of the patient and the presence or absence of other associated mechanical injuries.

Because the majority of burns in survivors of the Hiroshima attack were minor, little additional effect on mortality seemed to be caused by thermal injuries in those patients who suffered radiation injuries. However, based on results of experiments in animals, the combination of radiation and thermal injuries appears to cause a synergistic effect. Brooks et al.[14] found that the addition of 1 Gy of radiation increased the mortality in dogs with a 20-percent body surface area burn from 12 percent to 73 percent. Similar experiments in swine by Baxter et al.[15] demonstrated that 4 Gy of total-body radiation (which by itself causes 20-percent mortality) resulted in 90-percent mortality in animals with a 10-15-percent surface area burn that was otherwise nonlethal. In a rat study, Alpen and Sheline[16] found that the LA_{50} at 48 hours after thermal injury decreased from 32.8 percent to 23.9 percent when 5 Gy of radiation were added to the injury. Radiation doses of 1 Gy and 2.5 Gy, which by themselves were not lethal, markedly increased the mortality in a 30-percent burn model at 30 days. Based on these data, it is reasonable to assume that the combination of a radiation injury and a thermal burn (other than the most minor burn) will result in a mortality rate significantly higher than that expected from either injury alone. However, some levels of radiation injury and thermal injury will result in essentially 100-percent mortality by themselves, regardless of the presence or absence of any other injury.

Triage During Nuclear Warfare

After a nuclear attack, it is almost certain that sophisticated medical care of any type will be either severely limited or nonexistent. Triage, or sorting of casualties, is a system of evaluating or classifying casualties for the purpose of treatment. It is based on the principle of accomplishing the greatest good for the greatest number of wounded or injured individuals under the special circumstances present at a given time. Limits on available resources following a nuclear attack will clearly change the treatment recommendations for patients with thermal injuries and combined thermal-radiation injuries from those in a time of unlimited resources. During conventional warfare with limited resources, approximately 50 percent of young and middle-aged soldiers whose burns involve 60-70 percent of the total body surface area are saved.[17] Results are worse for those at the extremes of age. In this setting, expectant care should be applied to those patients with burns over more than 70 percent of their body surface area. Individuals with burns over less than 20 percent of their body surface area can usually have treatment delayed, and available resources can be applied to individuals with burns over 20-70 percent of their body surface area. As resources become more limited, the upper limit of the maximum size burn to be treated is decreased in 10-percent decrements until the patient load equals the resources available.

In the setting of nuclear attack, further restrictions in triage are inevitable. Individuals with thermal injury over less then 10 percent of the body surface area and no associated radiation or mechanical injury would be expected to survive without any significant treatment. Individuals with burns over more than 30 percent of the body surface area are unlikely to survive unless adequate treatment is available. Thus, when resources are limited it will be necessary to apply available resources to individuals who have thermal injury involving 10-30 percent of the body surface area. Because the exact effect of the combination of radiation and thermal injury on mortality in humans is unknown, it is impossible to give a definitive recommendation on treatment. Extremely minor thermal injury is unlikely to influence the mortality of radiation injury, and will not affect triage in this specific group. The presence of any identifiable symptoms of radiation injury in patients suffering a thermal injury over more than 30 percent of the body surface area will almost surely result in 100-percent mortality, unless extremely sophisticated resources are available. In an intermediate group, with thermal injury of 10-30 percent of the body surface area, one would expect a significant increase in mortality from a combination of thermal and radiation injury. In this group, the expenditure of health care resources should be decreased as the extent of burn and the dose of radiation increase.

Conclusions

Since the introduction of nuclear warfare in 1945, there have been significant improvements in burn care and corresponding decreases in mortality from burn injury. The large number of burn casualties following a nuclear attack on a population center will overwhelm available medical resources and make survival unlikely for anyone with a major burn injury. The exact effects of combined radiation and thermal injury in humans are undefined. At the extremes of injury, little effect will likely be noted. In the middle range of injury severity, a synergistic effect on mortality can be expected, based on experimental data.

References

1. *Burn Care Resources in North America, 1986-1987,* American Burn Association, St. Louis, MO, 1987.
2. Pruitt, B. A., Jr. The universal trauma model. *Bull Am Coll Surg* 70(10):2-13, 1985.
3. Pruitt, B. A., Jr. The burn patient: Initial care. In: *Current Problems in Surgery.* M. M. Ravitch, Ed., Year Book Medical Publishers, Chicago, 1979, pp. 5-61.
4. Reiss, E., Stirman, J. A., Artz, C. P., et al. Fluid and electrolyte balance in burns. *JAMA* 152:1309-1313, 1953.
5. Pruitt, B. A., Jr., and Curreri, P. W. The burn wound and its care. *Arch Surg* 103:461-468, 1971.
6. Tumbusch, W. T., Vogel, E. H., Jr., Butkiewicz, J. V., et al. Septicemia in burn injury. *J Trauma* 1:22-31, 1961.
7. Moncrief, J. A., Lindberg, R. B., Switzer, W. E., et al. Use of topical antibacterial therapy in the treatment of the burn wound. *Arch Surg* 92:558-565, 1966.
8. Herndon, D. N., and Parks, D. H. Comparison of serial debridement and autografting and early massive excision with cadaver skin overlay in the treatment of large burns in children. *J Trauma* 26(2):149-152, 1986.
9. Pruitt, B. A., Jr., and Levine, N. S. Characteristics and uses of biologic dressings and skin substitutes. *Arch Surg* 119:312-322, 1984.
10. Spebar, M. J. Medical aspects of nuclear warfare: A review. *Milit Med* 145(4):243-245, 1980.
11. Brode, H. L., and Small, R. D. A review of the physics of large urban fires. In: *The Medical Implications of Nuclear War.* National Academy Press, Washington, DC, 1986, pp. 73-95.
12. Postol, T. A. Possible fatalities from superfires following nuclear attacks in or near urban areas. In: *The Medical Implications of Nuclear War.* National Academy Press, Washington, DC, 1986, pp. 15-71.
13. Pruitt, B. A., Jr., Tumbusch, W. T., Mason, A. D., Jr., et al. Mortality in 1,100 consecutive burns treated at a burn unit. *Ann Surg* 159(3):396-401, 1964.
14. Brooks, J. W., Evans, E. I., Han, W. T., et al. The influence of external body radiation on mortality from thermal burns. *Ann Surg* 136(3):533-544, 1953.
15. Baxter, H., Drummond, J. A., Stevens-Newsham, L. G., et al. Reduction of mortality in swine from combined total body radiation and thermal burns by streptomycin. *Ann Surg* 137(4):450-455, 1953.

16. Alpen, E. L., and Sheline, G. E. Combined effects of thermal burns and whole body x irradiation on survival time and mortality. *Ann Surg* 140:113-118, 1954.
17. Department of Defense, *Emergency War Surgery*, 3rd edition. U.S. Government Printing Office, Washington, DC, 1988.

Complications of Combined Injury

Radiation Damage and Skin Wound Trauma in Mouse Models

G. David Ledney, Gary S. Madonna,
Daniel G. McChesney,
Thomas B. Elliott, and Itzhak Brook

Introduction

During nuclear disasters, most casualties will receive radiation of various energies, qualities, and doses. In addition, many individuals will die from combined injury, i.e., radiation plus burn and/or wound traumas. Judgments about medical care for casualties with combined injuries, such as those in the Chernobyl accident,[1] are difficult to make because clinical experience is limited, and data bases on relevant animal models are lacking. Investigators in our group are studying several complications of tissue trauma on irradiated mice to develop therapies for expected bacterial infections. Specifically, we are examining (1) the impact of radiation quality and type of injury on survival, (2) the effect of timing and extent of injury in combination with irradiation, (3) the hematopoietic responses after combined injury, and (4) the susceptibility of mice with combined injury to opportunistic and *Klebsiella pneumoniae* infections.

Materials and Methods

B6D2F1/J, B6CBF1/CUM, and C3H/HeN mice aged 12-20 weeks were used. The mice were quarantined on arrival and screened for disease before experimental use. They were maintained in an AAALAC-accredited facility in Micro-Isolator™ cages on hardwood chip bedding and provided with commercial rodent chow and acidified tap water *ad libitum*.

All injury procedures were done in compliance with guidelines from the National Research Council and the Armed Forces Radiobiology Research

G. D. LEDNEY, G. S. MADONNA, D. G. McCHESNEY, T. B. ELLIOTT, and I. BROOK, Experimental Hematology Department, Armed Forces Radiobiology Research Institute, Bethesda, Maryland 20814-5145.

Treatment of Radiation Injuries, Edited by
D. Browne *et al.,* Plenum Press, New York, 1990

Institute (AFRRI) committee on animal use and care. Mice were anesthetized by inhalation of methoxyflurane before tissue injury. Full-thickness, nonlethal skin injuries of various sizes were inflicted before or after irradiation by removing a section of the dorsal skin fold and underlying paniculous carnosus muscles with a steel punch.[2] The punch was immersed in 70-percent ethanol before each animal was injured. Burns were inflicted on the shaved dorsal surface area by a 12-s ignition of 95-percent ethanol.[3] After tissue trauma, all mice received 0.5 mL of 0.9-percent NaCl intraperitoneally (i.p.).

The techniques and dosimetry of irradiating mice in the AFRRI TRIGA reactor and cobalt-60 facilities were previously described.[4] All irradiations were performed at 0.4 Gy/min midline tissue by altering either experimental placement in the radiation field, reactor power, or shielding design. The desired neutron to gamma (n/γ) dose ratios were obtained by varying shielding configurations of lead, water, borated polyethylene, and paraffin at selected reactor powers. Mice were given bilateral exposures to cobalt-60 in aerated Plexiglas restrainers. Irradiation of mice in the reactor was done in aerated aluminum tubes that rotated at 1.5 rpm.

Results and Discussion

1. Survival of mice with combined injury depends on the quality and dose of radiation and the type of skin-wound injury.

Groups of B6D2F1 mice were irradiated with five different n/γ dose ratios produced by the TRIGA reactor. The n/γ dose ratios employed were 0.05, 0.33, 1, 3, and 19. Other groups of mice were irradiated with "pure" gamma radiation from a cobalt-60 source and the TRIGA reactor. Nonlethal 2.5-cm by 3.8-cm burns or wounds were inflicted 1 hour to 2 hours after each exposure, and 30-day survival responses were compared to control mice that were irradiated but uninjured. Thus, complete dose-response survival curves were obtained at each radiation quality with each type of injury. The radiation doses lethal to 50 percent of the mice in 30 days $(LD_{50/30})$ are presented in table 1. In all groups of mice, i.e., control irradiated, irradiated and burned, and irradiated and wounded, the $LD_{50/30}$ decreased as the proportion of neutrons in the total dose increased. At each n/γ dose ratio, postirradiation burn trauma and wound trauma reduced the $LD_{50/30}$ from the comparable radiation control group about 10 percent and 20 percent, respectively.

The time and frequency of mortality for irradiated animals reflect the organ system most severely damaged by radiation. That is, mice with severe intestinal cell damage die in about 7 days; mice with severe hematopoietic cell damage die in about 10-14 days. The intervals preceding death and the percentage of animals dying within those intervals are given in table 2 for the radiation qualities listed. The mortality percentages are based on a total of 30-60 mice

Table 1. Radiation Doses Required to Produce
50-Percent Lethality in Mice[1]

Radiation quality or n/γ dose ratio	Radiation dose (Gy)		
	Radiation only	Radiation and burn	Radiation and wound
Cobalt-60 (γ only)	9.65	8.20	7.61
TRIGA photons[2]	8.97	8.07	7.34
n/γ = 0.05	6.01	5.67	4.82
n/γ = 0.33	5.74	5.27	4.39
n/γ = 1	4.94	4.27	3.81
n/γ = 3	4.72	4.46	3.53
n/γ = 19	3.93	3.52	3.05

[1]All B6D2F1 mice were irradiated at 0.4 Gy/min, and $LD_{50/30}$ values were statistically determined from complete dose-response survival curves.
[2]Determination of the neutron dose is not possible using the paired ion chamber technique in this shield configuration. Based on activation foil analysis and neutron attenuation estimates, the neutron-to-gamma (n/γ) dose ratio was less than 0.01.

irradiated or with combined injuries at their respective $LD_{80/30}$ radiation doses. Most of the mice irradiated with an n/γ dose ratio of 19 died during the first week after exposure. Most of the mice exposed to the other radiation qualities died during the second postirradiation week. In animals with combined injuries (except cobalt-60-irradiated mice), 60 percent to 85 percent of irradiated and burned animals died 9-14 days after radiation exposure. Irradiation followed by wounding had the greatest impact on survival times: 80 percent to 95 percent of wounded mice given any quality of radiation died within 7-10 days after exposure.

The early mortality of mice irradiated with the high n/γ dose ratio may result from gastrointestinal tissue damage, because this proliferative epithelial cell system is sensitive to high fluxes of neutrons.[4] Thus, the absorptive ability and the protection afforded the host against subsequent translocation of intestinally derived bacteria are lost. The loss of the functional capacities of the intestinal system in mice results in death within 1 week.

In irradiated mice, skin wounding produces an open injury that is subject to evaporation of body water and to colonization of bacteria. In contrast, the burn site is covered by damaged but intact skin that may lessen the impact of water loss and bacterial colonization. Thus, the differences in $LD_{50/30}$'s and the mean time to death between irradiated-burned and irradiated-wounded mice may be explained by the nature of the injury sustained after exposure to radiation.

Table 2. Mortality of Irradiated Mice and Mice With Combined Injury, by Radiation Quality and Interval Between Radiation and Death

Interval (days)	Deaths (percent)				
	Cobalt-60	$n/\gamma = 0$[1]	$n/\gamma = 0.05$[1]	$n/\gamma = 1$[1]	$n/\gamma = 19$[1]
			Irradiated		
4-8	0	2.9	0	7.9	51.6
9-11	20.6	36.8	18.5	44.7	19.9
12-14	59.8	52.6	51.9	26.3	22.2
15-30	19.5	7.9	29.6	21.0	6.3
			Irradiated and burned		
4-8	31.0	3.0	27.8	25.6	3.3
9-11	17.2	51.5	16.7	34.9	63.3
12-14	13.7	36.4	50.0	27.9	20.0
15-30	37.9	9.1	5.5	11.6	13.3
			Irradiated and wounded		
4-8	67.9	54.5	36.7	69.2	75.6
9-11	28.5	31.8	43.3	17.3	4.8
12-14	3.6	9.4	10.0	7.7	7.3
15-30	0	0	10.0	5.8	12.2

[1]The n/γ represents neutron to gamma dose ratio.

2. Survival of mice with combined injury depends on the time of skin-wound injury relative to irradiation, the radiation dose, and the radiation quality.

In a series of studies, three groups of B6CBF1 mice were irradiated with three (9, 10, or 11 Gy) lethal doses of cobalt-60, respectively. At eight time points before irradiation and three time points afterward, 1.3-cm by 1.9-cm skin wounds were inflicted. The 30-day survival data are indicated in figure 1. Survival times of mice dying within that time frame (data not shown) were also recorded. The 30-day survival of animals wounded before irradiation increased as the time interval between injury and irradiation shortened. Further, the number of 30-day survivors increased when mice were wounded within 10 minutes after a nominally lethal radiation dose (9 Gy). The survival times of all control-irradiated mice that died within the 30-day period were 11-14 days. However, survival was extended to 17-20 days for mice irradiated with nominally lethal doses (9 Gy) when wounds were inflicted from 2 days before to 10 minutes after exposure. When wounds were inflicted 1 or 2 days after irradiation, the survival times for all groups of mice with combined injury were decreased to about 7 days.

In a second series of experiments, a comparative mortality study was done with B6D2F1 mice irradiated with sublethal doses of either cobalt-60 (7 Gy) or with an n/γ dose ratio of 19 (3 Gy). Groups of mice were injured at each

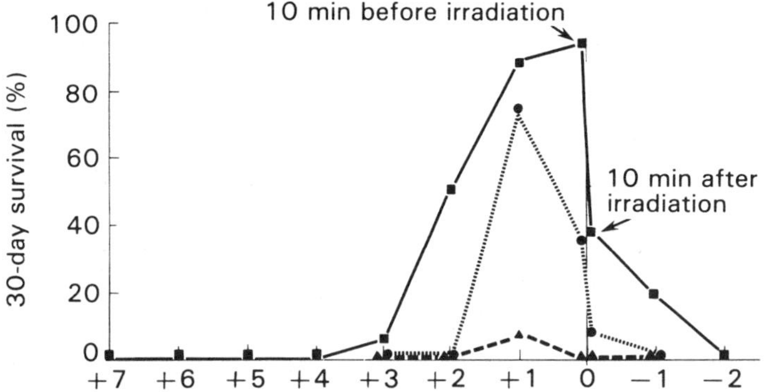

Day of wounding before (+) and after (−) cobalt-60 irradiation

Figure 1. Thirty-day survival of B6CBF1 female mice (n = 16/time point) after receiving 1.3-cm by 1.9-cm skin wounds and cobalt-60 irradiation. All control irradiated mice died; all control wounded mice lived; 9 Gy — ■ — ; 10 Gy ⋯ ● ⋯;11 Gy --▲--. (Previously published in *Experientia*, Volume 4, 1985.)

of three time points either before or after irradiation. The 30-day mortality data are shown in figure 2 and table 3. The incidence of death from combined injury was greater for animals irradiated with the high n/γ dose ratio (19) than with cobalt-60. In all irradiated mice, wound injury resulted in more deaths than burn injury. Burn or wound injury after irradiation resulted in more deaths than injuries given before exposure. As seen in the first series of experiments, injuries occurring shortly before (10 minutes) sublethal irradiation resulted in fewer mortalities than injuries inflicted 1 or 2 days before radiation exposure. In the second group of studies, a relatively similar decrease in mortality incidence was noted for animals injured soon after (10 minutes) irradiation compared to injuries inflicted 1 or 2 days later.

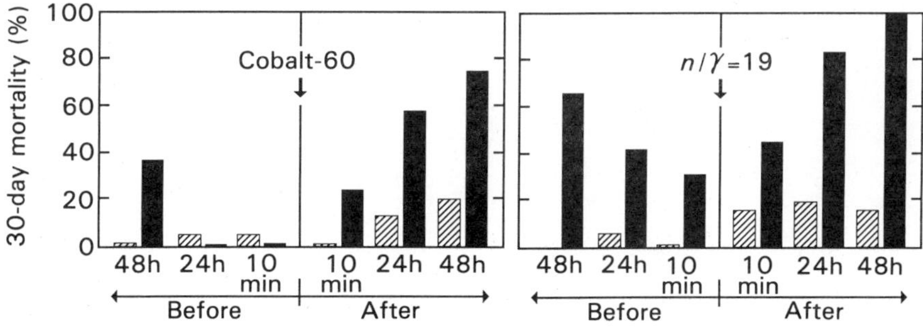

Time of injury relative to irradiation

Figure 2. Thirty-day mortality of B6D2F1 female mice after either 7 Gy cobalt-60 (n = 20/time point) or 3 Gy mixed field (n/γ = 19; n = 24/time point) irradiation and administration of 2.5-cm by 3.8-cm skin wounds ■ or skin burns ▨.

Table 3. Thirty-Day Mortality of Mice After
Combined Injury[1]

	Deaths/sample	
Injury	Cobalt-60 (7 Gy)	Mixed field $n/\gamma = 19$ (3 Gy)
Wound	1/36	4/100
Burn	2/36	4/100
Radiation	0/36	3/100

[1]Data reported for control mice only. B6D2F1 female mice received either cobalt-60 (n = 20/time point) or mixed-field radiation (n = 24/time point) and were administered 2.5-cm by 3.8 cm skin wounds or skin burns.

3. Skin-wound injury of irradiated mice stimulates hematopoiesis in restricted combined-injury situations.

As reported earlier, when the time interval between injury and irradiation is decreased, survival from combined injury may be increased when compared to cobalt-60-irradiated controls. In related experiments,[5] survival of mice recovering from irradiation correlated positively with increases in the number of endogenous colony-forming units found on the spleen (E-CFU-S). Quantification of E-CFU-S is a well-known measure of the undamaged hematopoietic proliferative potential of heavily irradiated mice. Thus, to determine if survival from combined injury positively correlated with increases in E-CFU-S, groups of B6CBF1 mice were irradiated with either 9, 10, or 11 Gy. Skin wounds (1.3 cm by 1.9 cm) were inflicted either 2 days, 1 day, or 10 minutes before irradiation, or 10 minutes or 1 day after irradiation. The mean values of 10-day E-CFU-S for 12-16 mice per treatment group are reported in table 4. A positive correlation was noted between the number of spleen colonies and survival from combined injury (figure 1). Thus, in restricted combined-injury situations, especially at nominally lethal radiation doses (9 Gy), trauma increased the hematopoietic proliferative compartments of irradiated mice.

Because trauma shortly after irradiation stimulated the hematopoietic proliferative cell compartment, the number of peripheral blood elements was determined. Thus, in a second series of hematopoietic studies, white blood cells, red blood cells, and platelets were determined in B6D2F1 mice inflicted with 2.5-cm by 3.8-cm injuries 1-2 hours after 7 Gy cobalt-60 irradiation. For nonirradiated, uninjured mice the blood cell numbers ($/mm^3$) were as follows: white blood cells, 4×10^3; red blood cells, 8×10^6; and platelets, 1×10^6. In 7-Gy-irradiated mice, the nadirs for the blood elements were as follows: white blood cells, 5×10^2 on day 14; red blood cells, 4.5×10^6 on day 14; and platelets, 2×10^5 on day 14. In mice with combined injury, nadir values similar to those

Table 4. Endogenous Colony-Forming Units-Spleen in Mice
After Wound Trauma and Irradiation

Cobalt-60 radiation dose (Gy)	Endogenous colony-forming units-spleen[1]					
	+2 days[2]	+1 day	+10 min	−10 min	−1 day	Irradiated only[3]
9.0	0.4±0.2	3.4±0.8	0.6±0.3	1.1±0.3	0	0
10.0	0.2±0.2	0.6±0.3	0	0	0	0
11.0	0	0.8±0.8	0	0	0	0

[1]All values = mean ± SE of 10 to 12 mice per group for spleen colonies counted 10 days after irradiation.
[2]The + = before irradiation, −= after irradiation.
[3]Irradiated controls had no endogenous colony-forming units-spleen. All mice died in irradiated control groups used for survival studies.

for irradiated mice were found, but at 7 days after exposure. Recovery in each blood cell type to 50 percent to 75 percent of nonirradiated, uninjured control values for mice with combined injury was on day 14 and day 21 for irradiated mice. Thus, injury of mice shortly after irradiation advances hematopoietic recovery by 1 week compared to irradiated animals.

4. Irradiation delays skin-wound closure in mice with combined injury; neutrons delay wound closure more than photons.

Wounding of irradiated mice increases the likelihood of death from bacterial infection because of (1) the colonization of the injury site with bacteria and (2) the associated granulocytopenia. Further, irradiation delays wound healing[6] and increases the risk for bacterial infection. The impact that radiation of different qualities has on skin-wound closure was examined in B6D2F1 mice inflicted with 2.5-cm by 2.5-cm skin wounds 1-2 hours after irradiation. Groups of 20 mice each were given either (1) 7 Gy cobalt-60, (2) 3.5 Gy with an n/γ dose ratio of 1, (3) 2.5 Gy with an n/γ dose ratio of 19, or (4) no radiation. These radiation doses are sublethal; neutron doses were chosen on the basis of a relative biological effect of 2 for n/γ = 1 and 2.8 for n/γ = 19 as determined in the $LD_{50/30}$ studies (table 1). Wound closure (100 mm^2) took place in 2 weeks for nonirradiated animals and 3 weeks for cobalt-60 irradiated mice (table 5). However, the wounds of mice given doses of neutrons closed 4 weeks after injury. Although the neutron doses are biologically equivalent to the cobalt-60 dose, these data suggest that neutrons induce more damage and/or impair repair processes in the skin epithelial cell-renewal system more than photons.

5. Resistance to exogenous bacterial challenge is dependent on radiation quality and may be enhanced by subsequent injury.

Table 5. Wound-Closure Times in Mice After Irradiation

Size of wound (mm^2)[1]	Days to the indicated wound size endpoint			
	$n/\gamma = 19$ (2.5 Gy)	$n/\gamma = 1$ (3.5 Gy)	Cobalt-60 (7 Gy)	Nonirradiated and wounded
300	19	16	13	7
100	27	27	21	12

[1]Two time points are given because eschar formation and retention prevented determination of full wound healing. The initial wound size was 625 mm².

In a series of studies, groups of B6D2F1 mice were irradiated with 7 Gy cobalt-60 or 3.5 Gy with an n/γ dose ratio of 1. On days 1, 4, 7, 10, and 14 after irradiation, mice were challenged subcutaneously with *Klebsiella pneumoniae*, and their survival was monitored for 30 days.[7,8] Groups of 8-20 mice were injected each day with bacteria doses of 10^1 to 10^6. The respective $LD_{50/30}$'s were statistically determined (table 6). Susceptibility of irradiated mice to challenge was greatest 4 days after exposure. At 10 days and 14 days after irradiation, neutron-irradiated mice were more resistant to challenge than mice given cobalt-60.

In a second group of bacterial susceptibility studies, B6D2F1 mice received 7 Gy of cobalt-60 and 2.5-cm by 3.8-cm wounds within 2 hours after irradiation. They were challenged with five different *K. pneumoniae* doses at the times indicated in the irradiated-mouse susceptibility studies. Because wounds were contaminated with several opportunistic bacteria and death followed, the

Table 6. $LD_{50/30}$ *K. Pneumoniae* Doses for Mice After Irradiation

Days of challenge after irradiation[1,2]	$LD_{50/30}$ *K. Pneumonia* doses	
	3.5 Gy $n/\gamma = 1$	7 Gy cobalt-60
1	8.51×10^2	8.51×10^2
4	6.46×10^1	2.89×10^2
7	2.76×10^4	8.51×10^3
10	1.29×10^5	4.27×10^2
14	1.91×10^6	4.48×10^4

[1]Mice were injected subcutaneously with *K. pneumoniae* and observed for 30 days. Each $LD_{50/30}$ value was statistically derived from the responses of at least five different bacterial doses; 8 to 20 mice were in each group.
[2]The $LD_{50/30}$ *K. pneumoniae* dose for nonirradiated mice ranges from 3×10^6 organisms to 9×10^6 organisms.

specific $LD_{50/30}$'s could not be determined. However, two observations were made. First, both mice with combined injury and those that were only irradiated were equally susceptible to subcutaneous *K. pneumoniae* challenge on days 1, 4, and 7 after irradiation. Second, mice with combined injury as a group were more resistant to challenge on day 10 (22 of 50 lived) and day 14 (38 of 50 lived) than mice that had been irradiated only (day 10, 13 of 50 lived; day 14, 17 of 50 lived). In another experiment, resistance to *K. pneumoniae* challenge 4 days after irradiation was greater in mice wounded 2 hours after exposure than in mice that had been irradiated only. The respective bacterial $LD_{50/30}$'s were 10^3 organisms and 10^2 organisms.

In these studies, wounding within 2 hours after irradiation appeared to confer resistance to subsequent exogenous bacterial challenge. The reason for this paradoxical finding is unclear, but it may stem from hematopoietic augmentation seen in mice with combined injury compared to lack of augmentation in mice given only radiation as reported in result 3.

6. Early mortality in mice with combined injury is associated with polymicrobic infections; ofloxacin therapy increases mean survival time.

Groups of C3H/HeN mice received (1) 8 Gy of cobalt-60 or (2) 8 Gy of cobalt-60 followed within 1 hour by a 1.3-cm by 1.9-cm skin wound. The mean survival times of mice in these treatment groups were 12.2 days and 5.5 days, respectively. Because of increased susceptibility to infection as a result of radiation-induced leukopenia and wounding, it was reasoned that the early death in mice with combined injury could be related to the unhindered spread of bacteria from the wound site and consequent sepsis and death. To test this hypothesis, mice were divided into groups—wounded mice, irradiated mice, and mice with combined injury—and euthanized on days 4, 5, 11, 12, 13, and 14. These time points preceded and/or included the days of death for groups with combined injury (days 4 and 5) and irradiated groups (days 11-14), respectively. On each of these days, the livers were removed and homogenized, and samples were cultured on bacteriological media. The wound sites of all injured mice were also cultured. On days 4 and 5, the liver cultures of irradiated mice and wounded mice yielded no bacterial growth, whereas liver cultures of mice with combined injury yielded *Streptococcus faecium*, *Staphylococcus aureus*, and *Escherichia coli*. These same organisms were also isolated from the wound cultures of these animals. *S. aureus* and *E. coli* were isolated from the livers of irradiated mice, but not until after day 11.

Because of the presence of polymicrobic infections in mice with combined injury 4 and 5 days after irradiation, we reasoned that aggressive antibiotic therapy might increase the survival time of these injured animals; no infection was detected in irradiated mice at that time. Although all mice died, treatment with the quinolone antibiotic ofloxacin increased the mean survival time of mice with combined injury from 5.5 days to 9.2 days. Significantly, in contrast to untreated mice with combined injury, no *E. coli* or other gram-negative bacilli were recovered from the wounds of these animals after only 1 day of treatment. Future studies that address infection will include the application of antiseptic to the wound site and combination therapy with synthetic trehalose dicorynomycolate (S-TDCM), an immunomodulator that increases nonspecific resistance to infection and stimulates hematopoiesis in irradiated animals.[7,8] Furthermore, because treatment with the antibiotic ofloxacin increases the mean survival time of mice with combined injury compared to that of irradiated mice, S-TDCM may be used to augment the undamaged hematopoietic proliferative potential of animals with combined injury.

Conclusion

Death from combined injury depends on the interaction between severe tissue injury induced by radiation and trauma and subsequent bacterial infections. Combined injury need not result in death if the extent of these injuries is reduced or modified by appropriate therapies. Indeed, residual reparative processes in proliferating cell renewal systems and antibacterial defenses exist in experimental models of lethal combined injury. It may be possible to augment these cell renewal and antibacterial systems with immunomodulating substances, in conjunction with therapy with new classes of antibiotics, such as the quinolones.

Acknowledgment

This work was supported by Armed Forces Radiobiology Research Institute, Defense Nuclear Agency, under Research Work Unit 00129. The views presented in this paper are those of the authors. No endorsement by the Defense Nuclear Agency has been given or should be inferred. Research was conducted according to the principles enunciated in the *Guide for the Care and Use of Laboratory Animals* prepared by the Institute of Laboratory Animal Resources, National Research Council.

References

1. Champlin, R. Treatment of victims of nuclear accidents: The role of bone marrow transplantation. *Radiat Res* 113:205-210, 1987.
2. Ledney, G. D., Stewart, D. A., Gruber, D. F., et al. Hematopoietic colony-forming cells from mice after wound trauma. *J Surg Res* 38:55-65, 1985.
3. Steritz, D. D., Bondi, A., McDermott, D., et al. A burned mouse model to evaluate anti-pseudomonas activity of topical agents. *J Antimicrob Chemother* 9:133-140, 1982.
4. Stewart, D. A., Ledney, G. D., Baker, W. H., et al. Bone marrow transplantation of mice exposed to a modified fission neutron (N/G 30:1) field. *Radiat Res* 92:268-279, 1982.
5. Ledney, G. D., Exum, E. D., Stewart, D. A., et al. Survival and hematopoietic recovery in mice after wound trauma and whole-body irradiation. *Exp Hematol* 10(Suppl 12):263-278, 1982.

6. Stromberg, L. W. R., Woodward, K. T., Mahin, D. T., *et al.* Combined surgical and radiation injury. The effect of timing of wounding and whole body gamma irradiation on 30 day mortality and rate of wound contracture in the rodent. *Ann Surg* 167:18-22, 1968.
7. Madonna, G. S., Ledney, G. D., Elliott, T. B., *et al.* Trehalose dimycolate enhances resistance to infection in neutropenic animals. *Infect Immun* 57:2495-2501, 1989.
8. McChesney, D. G., Ledney, G. D., and Madonna, G. S. Trehalose dimycolate enhances survival of fission neutron irradiated-mice and *Klebsiella pneumoniae*-challenged irradiated mice. *Radiat Res* 121:71-75, 1990.

Wound Environment

Implications for Healing and Infection

Patricia M. Mertz and William H. Eaglstein

Introduction

Recent advances in understanding the wound repair process have drawn attention to the complex series of events that follow injury. How the local wound environment can stimulate or retard regeneration and how environmental conditions can be controlled are reviewed in this chapter.

In the aftermath of a nuclear accident, patients with combined-injury wounds are a treatment challenge. Combined-injury wounds are defined as wounds from burns and/or trauma with local or systemic radiation exposure either before, during, or after the injuries. The wound-healing response in these patients is delayed because of their impaired immunological state and the synergistic characteristics of combined injury.[1]

This chapter presents the results of studies of acute wound and burn healing conducted in the model we developed for assessing epidermal repair and a discussion of occlusive dressings, matrix materials, and growth factors and their potential for wound healing.[2] This method for studying wound healing allows comparison of topical treatments in a relatively hairless animal, the domestic pig, which has skin similar to human skin.[3]

Materials and Methods

Young domestic pigs weighing 10-15 kg were conditioned for 2 weeks before the experiments. They were fed a basal swine diet *ad libitum* and housed individually with controlled temperature (19°-21°C) and on a 12-hour light/dark cycle. The conditions complied with requirements of the American

P. M. MERTZ and W. H. EAGLSTEIN, Department of Dermatology and Cutaneous Surgery, School of Medicine, University of Miami, Miami, Florida 33101.

Treatment of Radiation Injuries, Edited by
D. Browne *et al.,* Plenum Press, New York, 1990

Association for Laboratory Animal Science, and the studies were approved by the University of Miami Animal Research Committee.

Wounding Techniques and Treatment

Experimental animals were clipped with standard fine-tooth animal clippers. Skin on both sides of the animal was washed with a nonantibiotic soap (Neutrogena, Neutrogena Corporation, Los Angeles, CA). The animals were anesthetized with ketamine hydrochloride (i.m.) and inhalation of oxygen, halothane, and nitrous oxide.

Approximately 120-150 7-mm by 10-mm wounds were made 0.3 mm deep in the paravertebral and thoracic areas with an electrokeratome fitted with a 7-mm-wide razor blade to examine healing in partial thickness wounds.

Approximately 120 8.5-mm-diameter burns were made on the skin, anterior to the animals' coxal tuber to examine healing in burn wounds. An 8.5-mm-diameter brass rod weighing 358 g was heated to 100°C in a boiling water bath. The rod was placed for 6 seconds in a vertical position perpendicular to the skin surface with the pressure supplied by gravity. Immediately after the rod was removed, the burned epidermis was scraped off with a sterile spatula.

Partial-thickness wounds and burns were not studied in the same animal. Animals were divided into three groups so that a topical antibiotic, a vehicle, and air exposure could all be compared on the same animal. When dressing materials were examined in the model, wounds treated with dressings were compared to air-exposed controls.

Epidermal Migration Assessment

Beginning on day 2 or day 3 after keratome wounding and beginning on day 6 after burning, five or six partial-thickness wounds and the surrounding normal skin from each treatment group were excised with a standard width (22 mm) electrokeratome set to cut at a depth of 0.5 mm. On days 6-14, burn wounds were excised with the electrokeratome set to cut 0.6 mm deep. Specimens damaged during excision were discarded. Excised specimens containing the wound site were incubated in 0.5 M sodium bromide as described previously.[2] After incubation, dermis and epidermis were separated by placing the specimen epidermis side down on a glass slide and gently teasing the corner of the specimen with forceps to lift up the dermis. A glass slide was placed over the exposed epidermal edge to hold it in place. The entire dermis was pulled gently off the epidermis. The glass slide containing the epidermal specimen was placed on a cardboard sheet, and the epidermis was transferred to the cardboard with forceps so that the external part of the epidermis faced up. When crust was present in the wounded area on the epidermis, it was gently lifted away. The mounted epidermal sheet was examined macroscopically for defects (defined as holes in the epidermal sheet or as a lack of epidermal continuation in the area of the wound). Wounds were considered healed if there were no defects in the epidermis and considered not healed if there were defects.

Statistical Analysis

The number of wounds healed (epithelialized) was divided by the total number of wounds sampled per day and multiplied by 100. These data were used to construct a curve using the regression of logits versus log analysis time or probit analysis.[4] From these curves, the time needed for 50 percent of the specimens to be healed was estimated (healing time 50 = HT_{50}). To compare treatments, the relative rate of healing and the net relative rate of healing were calculated according to the following formulas:

Relative rate of healing = (HT_{50} control) - (HT_{50} treatment/HT_{50} control) x 100

Net relative rate of healing = (relative rate of active agent) - (relative rate of vehicle)

Statistical evaluation (x^2 using fourfold tables)[5] was performed on all animals from all treatment groups, starting with the day of initial healing. The day of initial healing for each animal was defined as the first day on which one or more of the sampled wounds showed complete healing. The purpose of tabulating data in this manner was to remove the variation in the overall healing response among animals.

Results and Discussion

The instant an injury occurs, a complex series of events begins, which in a healthy individual leads to tissue repair. The use of appropriate topical antiseptics and antimicrobials, dressing materials, electrical stimulation, matrix materials, or growth factors can stimulate tissue regeneration and may be especially important in combined injuries.

Antiseptics and Antimicrobials

The use of topical antiseptics and antimicrobials in wound care is based largely on tradition. Much of the data supporting their use has been anecdotal and their effects on wound healing are not well documented. Topical antimicrobials are used to reduce the number of bacteria contaminating wounds to prevent infection. However, it is important to remember that bactericidal agents that work on dry, intact skin may not be useful in wounded skin. For example, povidone-iodine (PI), an excellent antiseptic on intact skin, is not effective in wounds.[6] The antiseptic activity in the iodine is partly inactivated by proteins, wound fluids, and the bacteria in the wound itself.[7] A continuous supply of moist PI from a hydrogel has been shown to be effective for at least 24 hours;[8] however, there is controversy about its effect on skin cells, such as fibroblasts. Investigators who exposed fibroblasts in a tissue culture system to varying quantities of PI demonstrated that it was cytotoxic to fibroblasts.[9,10] It is difficult to know if these experiments approximate an *in vivo* wound situation because fibroblasts are actually grown in culture and then suspended in a bath of PI. It remains to be shown if PI used *in vivo* has the same effect. In studies that examined a daily application of PI to partial-thickness wounds in pigs, PI was shown to promote epidermal migration.[11]

Some antimicrobials have been shown to inhibit wound healing, and others have been shown to promote it (figures 1 and 2). Topical agents, which contain surfactants, may retard wound healing because of their formulation. Other topical antimicrobials may enhance epithelialization in addition to killing bacteria. Both Silvadine™ cream and Neosporin™ ointment have been shown to enhance epithelialization.[11] Many of these antimicrobial agents are in vehicles that enhance epidermal migration even before the active ingredients are added. Bactroban™, a new topical antimicrobial in a polyethylene glycol vehicle, has been shown to be neutral in animal wound-healing studies. The effect of Bactroban™ on impetigo is equal to that of oral erythromycin and dicloxacillin.[12,13] Topical Bactroban™ has a limited gram-negative spectrum and should be used with another agent if a mixed infection of gram-negative and gram-positive organisms is suspected.

Hibiclens® (chlorhexidine gluconate) is an effective antiseptic, but because it is extremely toxic to skin cells[14] its use as a wound cleanser is limited. It is toxic not only to the wound but also to health care personnel. Hibiclens® has been shown to cause keratitis and corneal opacity,[15] and should not be used on the face.

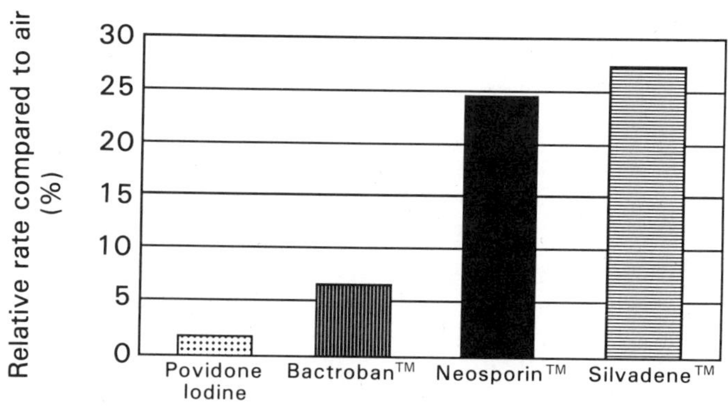

Figure 1. Antimicrobials that enhance epidermal migration.

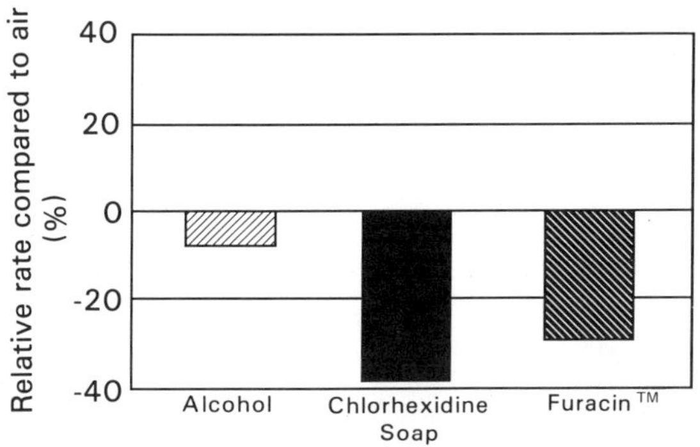

Figure 2. Antimicrobials that retard epidermal migration.

Dressing Materials

Occlusive wound dressings that stimulate wound healing while decreasing pain are now available (table 1). These new materials can protect the wound from pressure and exogenous bacterial pathogens, while maintaining a moist wound environment. The major mechanisms by which occlusive dressings stimulate healing are still not completely understood. Five possibilities[16] have been discussed: (1) easier migration of epithelial cells, (2) increased partial pressure of oxygen, (3) increased local concentration or availability of growth factors, (4) favorable effects of increased microbial flora, and (5) maintenance of an electrical potential between the wounded skin and surrounding normal skin.

Occlusive dressings can influence specific aspects of wound healing, and an optimal time for their use in acute wounds has been established. There is a "window" of time (between 6 hours and 24 hours) after wounding when the presence of an occlusive dressing produces an increased rate of resurfacing.[17] The dressings need to remain in place for at least 24 hours.[17] Occluded second-degree burn wounds in animals take twice as long to heal as excisional wounds of comparable depth. In our studies, burn-wound epithelialization was not enhanced by application of occlusive dressings.[18] Clinical investigations have shown that the moist wound environment created by these dressings has certain advantages; however, there is still controversy regarding their use because they stimulate not only healing but also the growth of bacteria.[19] Nevertheless, the fear of infection resulting from bacteria overgrowth has not been based on clinical experience.[20] On the contrary, few true infections have been associated with occlusive dressings, and the benefits to patient care far outweigh the failures. They not only promote healing but also reduce pain.[16]

Table 1. Advantages and Disadvantages of Various Occlusive Dressings

Dressing	Advantages	Disadvantages

Polyurethane films
OpSite®
Tegaderm®
Biocclusive®
	Transparent
	Moisture vapor
	   transmission
		May adhere to
		   friable skin

Hydrocolloids DuoDerm® J & J Ulcer Dressing®	Dressing material interacts with wound Wet to dry adherence	Opaque

Hydrogels
Vigilon®
Geliperm®
	Nonadherent
	Cooling
		Promotes gram-
		   negative
		   bacteria growth

Foams Synthaderm®	Nonadherent	Opaque
Laminates Biobrane®	Adherent Flexible	Opaque Allows exudate to escape

Animal studies have shown that some dressings provide wound protection from exogenous bacterial pathogens.[21] These dressings vary in composition, and no one material is appropriate for all wounds. The moisture-vapor transmission rates, adhesive qualities, and pressure-relief properties must be tailored to the location of the injury, the type of bacterial contamination present, and the condition of the surrounding normal skin. For example, wounds heavily contaminated with anaerobic organisms should be treated with dressings that allow atmospheric oxygen to come in contact with the wounds, so that anaerobic organisms will not proliferate.[22] An adhesive dressing should be used when noncompromised normal skin surrounds the wound. The nature of the adhesive on dressings makes stripping of normal skin stratum corneum likely, and can quickly lead to damage and breakdown of surrounding tissue.[23] Skin may be especially vulnerable in a trauma patient who has received radiation.

Wet to dry gauze should not be used on acute injuries because of the "reinjury effect." Reinjury is caused by removing dry gauze from a wound. Dry gauze removes newly formed epidermis as well as dead tissue, and harms delicate tissue, thereby delaying wound healing.[23]

Electrical Stimulation

Pulsed electrical stimulation has been shown to enhance epithelialization in animal wounds.[24] The amount of stimulation or retardation varies according to the polarity of the treatment electrode.[25] In addition to the effects on epidermis, pulsed electrical stimulation has been shown to influence dermal repair and, under certain conditions, to reduce wound fibroplasia significantly in humans.[26] Work is under way to miniaturize electrical devices for treating wounds. The prototypes will be programmable and contained in small, disposable adhesive bandages. When these are available, controlling scar formation may be possible. To our knowledge, use of these devices in treating burn injuries to prevent contracture has not been studied but is an area where research is needed.

Matrix Materials

Matrix materials are being developed that can replace dermal material and allow the ingrowth of fibroblasts to form new granulation tissue. The placement of bovine matrix materials in full-thickness wounds has reduced wound contracture.[27] These materials may support autografts or cultured epidermal cells to reform the entire missing skin. Work is under way to develop a skin substitute from matrix materials.

Growth Factors

Cell biologists are identifying proteins that are released shortly after injury and how they might be important to wound healing. The ability to generate large quantities of these proteins (regulatory peptides) through bioengineering has made it possible to treat wounds with them. Wound-healing studies using our animal model have demonstrated that topically applied recombinant human epidermal growth factor (rhEGF), basic fibroblast growth factor, recombinant human interleukin-1α (rhIL-1α), and transforming growth factor β can stimulate wound repair.[28-31] All these proteins are delivered from different vehicles into wounds and are either topically applied or injected into the wound site (table 2).

The importance of these growth factors in combined injuries has not been determined yet. Because the immunological status of individuals who receive combined injury is compromised, introduction of exogenous wound-healing growth factors may be especially important in treating combined injury.

Studies of acute wounds have demonstrated that vehicles not only are important as carriers of a substance but also play a role in determining the rate of growth-factor delivery from a vehicle.[32] For example, in laboratory studies, topical rhEGF was provided in two vehicles, a sustained release vehicle and a pulsed release vehicle. Both treatments were placed on animal wounds twice a day. The EGF pulsed release vehicle system was found to be more effective for stimulating epithelialization.[28]

Table 2. Growth Factors Evaluated in the Porcine Model

Factor	Investigator	Dose	Type of wound	Relative rate of healing (percent)
RhEGF	Mertz et al.[28]	25 μg/mL[T] twice a day (days 0-6)	Partial thickness	13
Basic FGF	Hebda et al.[29]	10 μg/wound[T] once, day 0	Partial thickness	21
rhIL-1α	Mertz et al.[30]	4.0 μg/site[T] daily (days 0-6)	Partial thickness	29
rhIL-1α	Mertz et al.[30]	40 μg/site[I] daily (days 0-6)	Partial thickness	2
TGFβ	Hebda[31]	60 μg[I] once, day 0	Partial thickness	0
TGFβ	Hebda[31]	60 μg[I] once, day 0	Second-degree burn	4

T, topical.
I, injected.
RhEGF, recombinant human epidermal growth factor.
FGF, fibroblast growth factor.
rhIL-1α, recombinant human interleukin 1α.
TGFβ, transforming growth factor β.

Addition of exogenous IL-1α in a water-based cream has been shown to stimulate epithelialization of partial-thickness wounds in pigs. In addition, porcine keratinocytes have high-affinity binding sites for recombinant human IL-1α.[30] Dose-response studies currently are being conducted. The role of IL-1α on burn-wound healing remains to be determined.

Conclusion

Wound environments can be manipulated to enhance acute wound and burn healing, but it remains to be seen if the same premises and modalities apply to combined injury. It is possible that wound-healing response following combined injury is significantly different from the healing response following the injuries that have been studied. Definitive investigations of combined-injury wound healing should be undertaken.

References

1. Oughterson, A. W., and Warren, S. *Medical Effects of the Atomic Bomb in Japan, Vol. 8.* National Nuclear Energy Series. Division VIII. Vol. 8. McGraw-Hill Book Company, Inc., New York, 1956.
2. Eaglstein, W. H., and Mertz, P. M. New method for assessing epidermal wound healing: The effect of triamcinolone acetonide and polyethylene film occlusion. *J Invest Dermatol* 71(6):382-384, 1978.
3. Winter, G. D. Formation of scab and the rate of epithelialization on superficial wounds in the skin of domestic pig. *Nature* 193:293-294, 1964.
4. Zar, J. H. *The Normal Distribution in Biostatistical Analysis.* Prentice-Hall, Englewood Cliffs, New Jersey, 1974.
5. Armitage, P. *Statistical Methods in Research.* Blackwell Scientific Publications, Oxford, 1971, pp. 131-134.
6. Mertz, P. M., Alvarez, O. M., Smerbeck, R. V., et al. A new *in vitro* model for the evaluation of topical antiseptics on superficial wounds: The effect of 70% alcohol and povidone-iodine solution. *Arch Dermatol* 120:58-62, 1984.
7. Ulrich, J. A. Antimicrobial efficacy in the presence of organic matter. In: *Skin Microbiology Relevance to Clinical Infections.* H. Maibach and R. Aly, Eds. Springer Verlag, New York, 1981, pp. 149-157.
8. Mertz, P. M., Marshall, D. A., and Kuglar, M. A. The effect of povidone iodine in polyethylene oxide hydrogel dressing on multiplication of *Staphylococcus aureus* in partial-thickness wounds. *Arch Dermatol* 122:1133-1138, 1986.
9. Rodeheaver, G., Bellamy, W., Kody, M., et al. Bactericidal activity and toxicity of iodine-containing solutions in wounds. *Arch Surg* 117:181-185, 1982.
10. Pratt, L., Balin, A. K., and Carter, D. M. Dilute povidone-iodine solutions inhibit human fibroblast growth. *J Clin Res* 33:676, 1985.
11. Geronemus, R. G., Mertz, P. M., and Eaglstein, W. H. Wound healing: The effects of topical antimicrobial agents. *Arch Dermatol* 115:1311-1314, 1979.
12. Mertz, P. M., Dunlop, B. W., and Eaglstein, W. H. The effects of Bactroban™ ointment on epidermal wound healing in partial thickness wounds. In: *Bactroban (Mupirocin). Proceedings of an International Symposium.* R. L. Dobson, J. J. Leyden, W. C. Noble, et al., Eds. Excerpta Medica, Princeton, 1985, pp. 211-215.
13. Mertz, P. M., Marshall, D. A., Eaglstein, W. H., et al. Topical mupirocin treatment of impetigo is equal to oral erythromycin therapy. *Arch Dermatol* 125:1069-1073, 1989.
14. Lineweaver, T. Topical antimicrobial toxicity. *Arch Surg* 120:267-270, 1985.
15. Hamed, L. M., Ellis, F. D., Boudreault, G., et al. Hibiclens keratitis. *Am J Ophthalmol* 104:50-56, 1987.
16. Eaglstein, W. H. Experiences with biosynthetic dressings. *J Am Acad Dermatol* 12:434-440, 1985.
17. Eaglstein, W. H., Davis, S. C., Mehle, A. L., et al. Optimal use of an occlusive dressing to enhance healing. *Arch Dermatol* 124(3):392-395, 1988.
18. Davis, S. C., Mertz, P. M., and Eaglstein, W. H. The effects of DuoDerm® and Opsite®, two occlusive dressings, on second-degree burn wound healing. *J Invest Dermatol* 86(4):470 (Abstract), 1986.
19. Mertz, P. M., and Eaglstein, W. H. The effect of a semi-occlusive dressing on the microbial population in superficial wounds. *Arch Surg* 119:287-289, 1984.
20. May, S. R. Physiology, immunology and clinical efficacy of an adherent polyurethane wound dressing: OpSite®. In: *Burn Wound Coverings. Vol. II.* D. L. Wise, Ed. CRC Press, Boca Raton, Florida, 1984, pp. 53-78.
21. Mertz, P. M., Marshall, D. A., and Eaglstein, W. H. Occlusive wound dressings to prevent bacterial invasion and wound infection. *J Am Acad Dermatol* 12(4):662-668, 1985.

22. Marshall, D. A., Mertz, P. M., and Eaglstein, W. H. An evaluation of the multiplication of some common pathogens in wounds treated with various occlusive dressing. *J Invest Dermatol* 86(4):492 (Abstract), 1986.
23. Alvarez, O. M., Mertz, P. M., and Eaglstein, W. H. The effect of occlusive dressings on collagen synthesis and reepithelialization in superficial wounds. *J Surg Res* 35(2):142-148, 1981.
24. Davis, S. C., and Mertz, P. M. The effect of pulsed electrical stimulation on epidermal wound healing. *J Invest Dermatol* 90(4):555 (Abstract), 1988.
25. Davis, S. C., Cazzaniga, A., Reich, J. D., et al. Pulsed electrical stimulation: The effect of varying polarity. *J Invest Dermatol* 92:418 (Abstract), 1989.
26. Weiss, D. S., Eaglstein, W. H., and Falanga, V. Pulsed electrical stimulation decreases scar thickness at split-thickness graft donor sites. *J Invest Dermatol* 92:539 (Abstract), 1989.
27. Alvarez, O. M. Cultured epidermal autografts in clinics in dermatology. In: *Clinics in Dermatology*. W. H. Eaglstein, Ed. J. B. Lippincott, Philadelphia, 1984, pp. 54-67.
28. Mertz, P. M., Davis, S. C., Arakawa, Y., et al. Pulsed rhEGF treatment increased epithelialization of partial thickness wounds. *J Invest Dermatol* 90:588 (Abstract), 1988.
29. Hebda, P. A., Klingbeil, C., Abraham, J., et al. Acceleration of epidermal wound healing by human basic fibroblast growth factor. *J Invest Dermatol* 90:568 (Abstract), 1988.
30. Mertz, P. M., Davis, S. C., Eaglstein, W. H., et al. Interleukin-1 is a potent inducer of wound reepithelialization. *J Invest Dermatol* 92:480 (Abstract), 1989.
31. Hebda, P. A. The acceleration of epidermal wound healing in partial thickness burns by transforming growth factor-beta. *J Invest Dermatol* 92:442 (Abstract), 1989.
32. Eaglstein, W. H., and Mertz, P. M. "Inert" vehicles do affect wound healing. *J Invest Dermatol* 74:90-91, 1980.

Combined Injury Complications

Roundtable Discussion
(Questions and discussions were summarized by the book editors.)

Question:

Would an irradiated patient with burns or other combined injuries benefit from bone marrow transplantation?

Discussion:

The crux of the question is, What is the probability of death from bone marrow failure? If the irradiated patient is going to die of skin burns, transplantation or any amount of therapy is irrelevant. But if the physician does not know if the patient will die of skin burns, the physician must decide if the bone marrow is to be reconstituted. The probability of death from hematopoietic failure versus the risk/benefit ratio of various therapies must be calculated. If the therapy is to have a low-risk/high-benefit ratio, as does the transfusion of irradiated red blood cells, then the treatment should be given. If hematopoietic growth factors are to be used, the risk/benefit ratio is not as certain—it is possible that giving hematopoietic growth factors can make the situation worse as well as better. For example, if the patient has internal contamination with radioactive cesium, as in Goiânia, hematopoietic cells may be exposed to ongoing radiation.

When transplanting marrow, the risk/benefit ratio is less clear, because new stem cells may be needed, and graft-versus-host disease may develop. There is a data base of about 8,000 patients who have received bone marrow transplants, but there is no simple answer. With each radiation victim, the probability of death from bone marrow failure and the likelihood of success of therapeutic intervention in that patient is calculated. If a person who is exposed to radiation is less than 20 years old, the probability of success of the transplant is about twice as high as in a person older than 40. If the donor is an HLA-identical sibling, the probability of benefiting from transplantation is 2-3 times greater than if the donors are mismatched. If the victim is 6 years old and has a genetically identical twin, a bone marrow transplant will be done because the benefit/risk ratio is favorable. If the victim is a 75-year-old man and has a completely mismatched female daughter, a bone marrow transplant will not be done, and there is nothing magical nor are there any more general principles that can be applied. The question about skin burns or other injuries is irrelevant because bone marrow transplants can only correct hematopoietic failure. For example, transplants cannot correct interstitial pneumonia from inhaled radioactive particles.

Question:

Using a risk/benefit ratio, how would the presence of a sublethal but significant burn, say a 10-15 percent full-thickness burn, affect the decision to do a transplant?

Discussion:

If there is uncertainty whether the patient will survive a nonhematopoietic injury, the hematopoietic injury should be assessed with varying risk/benefit ratios. If the patient has received less than approximately 8 Gy, a bone marrow transplant may not be needed. If the patient received more than 8 Gy, a transplant should be done. If the patient received more than 8 Gy and has a genetically identical twin, the patient should get a bone marrow transplant from the twin. With a dosage of more than 10 Gy, the patient will probably get a transplant because there is no possibility of recovery without it. Physicians will transplant 100 people knowing that 80 will die of burns to save the 20, because if the physicians have to wait to see who the 80 are that are going to die of burns, they will no longer be able to rescue the 20. All the Chernobyl victims who the treating physicians thought would die of burns did not, and all those who were predicted to die from hematopoietic injury did not die either. It is a guessing game.

In mouse models of combined injury, bone marrow was transplanted to obtain survival data on lethally irradiated mice and injured mice. The experimental plan was to use three different doses of radiation: (a) a nominally lethal dose, (b) a lethal dose plus 1 Gy, and (c) a lethal dose plus 2 Gy. Syngeneic bone marrow transplantation (where the animal donor and recipient are genetically similar) was performed to answer the question, Is survival after lethal irradiation and subsequent wound trauma dependent on the number of surviving bone marrow cells? Wound trauma was inflicted 1-2 hours after irradiation, and animals were treated 1 day later with 1×10^5 bone marrow cells (a dose that rescues lethally irradiated mice) and 4×10^7 bone marrow cells. In this discrete experiment, neither dose of bone marrow cells rescued any animals subjected to the three doses of radiation in combination with wound trauma.

Question:

What are some distinctions between thermal burns and radiation burns?

Discussion:

The distinction between thermal burns and radiation burns is significant, especially in surgical management. In general, thermal burns can be seen, are self-limited, and if excised, they are gone. The leg injuries shown in the photographs of the San Salvador patient cannot be called burns in the traditional sense of the word, and they require therapy that is far different from thermal burn treatment. Whereas treatment of thermal burns involves early excision and skin grafting, the radiation burn requires long-term surgical management.

Although we have reached a consensus about treating radiation burns and thermal burns differently, no one has described these differences. Treatments for thermal burns have been known and practiced for some time. A point was made that it is important to treat radiation burns early, especially burns that involve damage to the vasculature, when there is extensive total-body exposure. When patients with radiation burns become immunosuppressed and pancytopenic, it is much more difficult to achieve closure. It is also important to close the wound as soon as possible to prevent infection. Specific management skills or techniques that differ in treating thermal burns and radiation burns should be addressed in detail in another forum.

Question:

What are the recommendations for antibiotic therapy for burn patients who would likely be febrile 24 hours after injury and patients with multiple trauma where fever is an expected variable during the course of the disease?

Discussion:

Antibiotic therapy should be started early, possibly even on day 0, based on animal data showing that wounds will colonize early. For the patient who has no associated injuries (only has radiation injuries), the patient should be febrile and neutropenic before starting antibiotics.

A distinction should be made between infections associated with burns and infections associated with other trauma. Infections with burns can occur immediately or 3 weeks later. In the beginning, *staphylococcus* or other skin-inhabitant infections are problems, whereas later *pseudomonas* can become a problem. The types of antibiotics necessary in the early postirradiation period and those needed during the late postinjury period must be defined. Timing is important.

Question:

When patients have severe burns and require surgery within the first few days after irradiation, what are the recommendations for prophylactic and therapeutic antibiotics?

Discussion:

Antibiotics should not be used empirically. The only data that indicate some advantage or some validity for using antibiotics in surgery are reported in the prevention of wound infections. There are no data to support less intraperitoneal sepsis or fewer abscesses by using perioperative, intraoperative, or postoperative antibiotic therapy. The only reason for using antibiotics is to control wound sepsis. In nonirradiated patients, sepsis can be controlled in other ways, for example, by leaving the wound open. Ideally, antibiotics should not be used unless there is a septic source or you operate on a patient who is already bacteremic or septicemic.

Question:

Is the patient who requires invasive catheters and plastic tubes, for example, considered a patient with combined injuries because we know these devices have a high likelihood of colonizing bacteria and infecting the patients?

Discussion:

Catheters placed in hospitalized neutropenic or leukemic patients may become colonized. If antibiotics are started early as a routine general hygiene measure, there is likely going to be colonization with resistant organisms, and more likely, the patient will become colonized with *candida*. Generally, treat the febrile, neutropenic patient empirically. Do not initiate a broad spectrum combination in a neutropenic but otherwise stable patient without signs of infection. The patient with multiple injury is the most complex to treat; treatment is really a judgment call. But, treatment for the patient who has been exposed to high doses of radiation and is expected to become neutropenic generally does not include therapeutic antibiotics. The patient should be observed carefully and, at the first sign of fever, antibiotics should be initiated.

Question:

In animal models, Aquaphor enhances epithelialization. What has been the experience in using Aquaphor for the treatment of burn victims in radiation accidents?

Discussion:

The Mexican physicians selected Aquaphor for the treatment of the Salvadorian patients. Surprisingly, the two men, who would have been expected to be in severe pain from these lesions, did not experience much foot pain, and required little drug intervention for pain. It is unclear whether Aquaphor was used to treat the Chernobyl victims because the name brands of many preparations in the U.S.S.R. are different.

Question:

What are some of the issues concerning triage of patients with combined injury after various types of radiation accidents or incidents?

Discussion:

Studies using animal models of combined injury and data from the Chernobyl accident suggest that there is a much higher mortality rate in patients with combined injury. During triage of many casualties, the physician might decide not to provide care to those with combined injuries who are not likely to survive, but rather use the minimal resources available to treat those who are likely to survive, for example, patients with limited combined injury, trauma only, or radiation exposure only.

During triage, some idea of dosimetry is needed, particularly in the military environment. The military expect to soon have physical dosimeters in the field. Military personnel will wear wrist dosimeters that will quantify both neutrons and photons, and will give medical personnel information on doses of radiation that can be invaluable in making decisions about who should be treated.

We considered the temporality of traumatic, burn, and radiation injuries in the definition of combined injury, that is, not having recovered from one injury before another is added. Considering the dynamics of the patient, the outcome can vary depending on the sequence of injury or insult. Animal experiments suggest that slight wounds before irradiation can stimulate hematopoiesis, producing a radioprotective effect. A neutropenic patient who has been in a fallout field has a compromised hematopoietic system, then receives a wound, will be in worse shape than a nonneutropenic wounded patient.

We do not fully understand all the nuances of treatment in the patient with combined injury. For example, we do not know the effectiveness of the immunomodulators, how much and when to give antibiotic therapy, or the role of blood products. Whether we should be more aggressive with some antibiotic therapy or use higher doses to compensate for the decreased immunity is not clear. For example, if we treat too aggressively with an antibiotic for trauma, the patient may die sooner from the infection due to irradiation.

Future Directions
and
Consensus Summary Statement

A Historical Perspective on the Therapy
of Total-Body Radiation Injury

Eugene P. Cronkite

Introduction

A brief look at previous research will show how we arrived where we are today. Shielding and transplantation of bone marrow were initiated long ago. In 1912, Chiari[1] demonstrated that bone marrow of the rabbit grew when transplanted into the spleen only when the spleen was shielded from irradiation. Fabricius-Moller[2] showed in 1922 that shielding portions of the skeleton prevented a decline in the number of blood platelets and consequently prevented radiation hemorrhage. In 1951, Jacobson et al.[3] attained nearly 100-percent protection from lethal doses of radiation when the mouse spleen was shielded. In 1951, Brecher and Cronkite[4] showed that shielding of one parabiotic rat protected the other rat from fatal irradiation. These studies clearly demonstrated that protecting the spleen of the mouse or the bone marrow of the guinea pig prevented the sequelae of marrow aplasia, and that some protective substance or cells circulated from the nonirradiated parabiont to the irradiated parabiont. Lorenz et al.[5] proved in 1952 that the protection was from cells located in the bone marrow or spleen, because one could protect mice from lethal irradiation by transfusing marrow cells or spleen cells in the mouse. Ford et al.[6] proved in 1956, by using a marker chromosome, that transplantation of donor hematopoietic cells had occurred.

Clinicians have long known that marked granulocytopenia predisposes patients to bacterial infections, either from pathogens or from commensal organisms with which the individual usually lives in harmony. Evidence that infection was of major importance was obtained from (1) clinical observations of bacterial infection in human beings exposed to atomic bomb radiation in Hiroshima and Nagasaki, in reactor accidents, and in large animals dying from radiation exposure; (2) correlative studies on mortality rate, time of death, and incidence of positive culture in animals; (3) studies of irradiated animals challenged with normally nonvirulent organisms; (4) studies of germ-free mice

---

E. P. CRONKITE, Medical Department, Brookhaven National Laboratory, Upton, New York 11973.

Treatment of Radiation Injuries, Edited by
D. Browne *et al.*, Plenum Press, New York, 1990

and rats; and (5) studies of the effectiveness of antibiotics in reducing mortality rates. The foregoing observations were covered in detail in 1969 by Bond, Cronkite, and Conard.[7]

General knowledge and sound experimental data on animals and humans clearly demonstrate that the sequelae of pancytopenia (bacterial infection, thrombocytopenic hemorrhage, and anemia) are the lethal factors. Much research was required to demonstrate that there were no mysterious radiation toxins, that hyperheparinemia was not a cause of radiation hemorrhage, and that radiation hemorrhage could be prevented by fresh platelet transfusions.[8]

Classic Syndromes Produced by Uniform Total-Body Radiation

Radiation syndromes produced by exposure to ionizing radiation are dependent on the total dose, the energy of the radiation, and the ensuing depth-dose patterns.* Three somewhat arbitrary and overlapping syndromes are the central nervous system (CNS) syndrome, gastrointestinal (GI) syndrome, and hematopoietic syndrome.

CNS Syndrome

The CNS syndrome occurs after large doses of several thousand cGy. Death may occur during exposure in some laboratory animals. Death is preceded by hyperexcitability, ataxia, respiratory distress, and intermittent stupor. Doses capable of producing this syndrome are uniformly fatal. Because it is highly unlikely that a methodology will be developed to reverse the necrotizing of brain lesions, this is not a fertile area for investigation.

GI Syndrome

The GI syndrome is produced by a wide range in doses (2-20 Gy). Doses in excess of 10 Gy are fatal within 3-9 days in laboratory animals and probably in humans as well. The GI syndrome is characterized by marked nausea, vomiting, diarrhea, and denudation of the small bowel mucosa. Severe and persistent GI syndrome was observed in Japan and described by Oughtersen and Warren[9] and in some accidents by Hubner and Fry.[10] Brecher et al.[11] prolonged the life of dogs exposed to 12 Gy by intensive administration of intravenous fluids and plasma. Treated dogs that survived doses of up to 12

---

*The dose unit used is the Gy, a physical dose unit equal to 10^4 erg/gram in tissue. It is independent of quality of radiation (linear energy transfer). The Gy equals 100 rad, an older radiation dose unit; 1 cGy equals 1 rad.

Gy regenerated the mucosa of the small intestine within 6 days.[11] Survivors of this syndrome then experienced the sequelae of marrow depression. The GI and hematopoietic syndromes were observed in the Japanese exposed in Hiroshima and Nagasaki.[9] Because the GI syndrome is due to failure of timely renewal of the GI epithelium, a probable area of profitable research would be to search for unknown molecular regulators or to apply known regulators that control steady-state self-renewal in the GI tract to accelerate the repletion of the GI tract.

Hematopoietic Syndrome

The hematopoietic syndrome is not necessarily fatal. It occurs in the range of 1.5-8 Gy in all mammals, including humans, and is usually preceded by transient nausea, vomiting, and diarrhea lasting a few hours or days. Clinical hematologists have long been familiar with management of granulocytopenia, thrombocytopenia, and anemia with bacterial infection and purpura. The hematopoietic syndrome presents no mysteries to the practicing hematologist and oncologist. The only question is, When should one transplant marrow?

Radiation Injury in Hiroshima and Nagasaki

The CNS syndrome was not observed by the Japanese in Hiroshima and Nagasaki, nor would one have expected it to be, because doses of the size that produce the syndrome occurred well within the area of total destruction. The GI syndrome with death in the first week was well documented clinically and pathologically.[9] The sequence in depletion of blood counts is different in humans and animals; it takes longer for the hematopoietic syndrome to develop in humans. For example, deaths from infections were most prevalent in the second through fourth weeks (maximum incidence during the third week) and from hemorrhagic phenomena during the third to sixth weeks (maximum incidence in the fourth week). Deaths from radiation hemorrhage and infection occurred in the Japanese as late as the seventh week, in contrast with animals, in which deaths were uncommon later than the thirtieth day. The neutrophil count after irradiation has been correlated with mortality in animals exposed to bomb gamma radiation at the Pacific Proving Ground and also in the Japanese in Hiroshima and Nagasaki.[12] The neutrophil count is probably the best clinical sign of severity of injury.[13]

Survival After Total-Body Irradiation

After studying the report by the Joint Commission on the Effects of the Atomic Bomb in Japan and the analysis by Oughtersen and Warren,[9] I proposed in 1957 that there are three types of survival groups based on signs and symptoms: survival improbable, survival possible, and survival probable.[14]

Survival Improbable

Vomiting occurs promptly or within a few hours and continues, followed in rapid succession by prostration, diarrhea, anorexia, and fever. Death will probably occur in 100 percent of these individuals within the first week unless they receive extensive symptomatic therapy.

Survival Possible

Vomiting may occur but is of relatively short duration, followed by a period of well-being. In this period of well-being, marked changes take place in the hematopoietic tissues. Lymphocytes are profoundly depressed within hours and remain so for months. The neutrophil count falls to low levels. The degree and time of maximum depression depends on the degree of radiation injury (as described by Jacobs *et al.*).[12]   Signs of bacterial infection may develop when the neutrophil count falls below 0.5×10^9/L. Probability of infection is increased by burns and open wounds. Platelet counts may reach very low levels within 2 weeks. Bleeding may occur within 2-4 weeks. The survival-possible group represents the lethal dose range in the classical pharmacological sense. The latent period lasts from 1-3 weeks with little clinical evidence of injuries other than slight fatigue. At the end of the latent period, the patient may develop purpura, epilation, cutaneous ulcerations, infections of wounds or burns, diarrhea, and/or melena. With therapy of antibiotics and/or sulphonamides and platelet transfusions, the survival time and rate can be expected to increase.

In Japan, many soldiers had nausea and vomiting; recovered and felt well; returned to duty; later developed purpura, epilation, and cutaneous lesions; and then died of infections. This pattern was well documented by Oughtersen and Warren.[9] The data of Kikuchi and Wakisaka[15] indicate that granulocytes decreased more rapidly in individuals who could be assigned to the survival-improbable and survival-possible groups than in those in the survival-probable group. Fliedner *et al.*[13] have extensively analyzed human radiation injury cases, correlating survival with changes in the peripheral granulocytes and platelet counts and developing a computer model for predicting the probability of survival. Research should continue on correlating data on hematologic response with probability of survival.

The recent research of Storb *et al.*[16] on dogs suggests that matched bone marrow transplantation is probably indicated in the survival-possible group, because dogs exposed to varying doses of radiation will reject the marrow if it is not needed and accept it if required for lifesaving restoration of aplastic marrow. Graft-versus-host disease will develop in a variable fraction of transplanted individuals. A clinical axiom states that it is better to have a live ailing patient on your hands than a cadaver. The survival-possible group may benefit substantially from the judicious administration of the now-available molecular hematopoietic growth factors. Extensive clinical and animal research is required to develop the best methods of using these agents to accelerate regeneration of hematopoiesis and/or regeneration of transplanted bone marrow.

Survival Probable

This group consists of individuals who may or may not have had nausea, vomiting, and diarrhea on the day of exposure. For example, a quarter of the Marshallese had nausea and vomiting.[17] Many Japanese had significant depression of leukocytes and platelets but no clinical sequelae of bone marrow depression. If there has been no GI symptomatology, the only way to detect individuals in this group is to perform serial studies on the blood, with particular reference to granulocytes, lymphocytes, and platelets. The lymphocytes may reach a low constant level early, within 48 hours of exposure, and show little evidence of recovery for many months thereafter.

Granulocytes may show some depression during the second and third weeks. A late fall in granulocytes during the sixth and seventh weeks after exposure may be observed. Platelet counts reach the lowest levels at approximately the thirtieth day—the time when maximum bleeding was observed in the Japanese exposed at Hiroshima and Nagasaki. Lowest platelet counts were also seen in the Marshallese exposed to fallout radiation about 30 days after exposure.[17] Individuals with neutrophil counts below $1 \times 10^9/L$ may be asymptomatic. Likewise, individuals with platelet counts of $75 \times 10^9/L$ or less may show no external signs of bleeding. Individuals in this group do not need treatment. Radiation doses, for reasons to be discussed later, may be misleading and are not helpful. It is known from the studies in Japan that after exposure to 2 Gy (a sublethal dose of radiation), the incidence of leukemia increased about 10 percent. Theoretically, one could argue that individuals exposed to doses of radiation that increase the incidence of leukemia, such as 0.5 Gy or more, should not receive hematopoietic molecular regulators to accelerate regeneration, because premature stimulation of initiated cells may fix a lesion in DNA conducive to the later development of leukemia, possibly increasing the late incidence of leukemia or decreasing the latency.

Further research is needed to determine (in animal models) whether the administration of hematopoietic molecular regulators, for example, granulocyte colony-stimulating factor (G-CSF), will force initiated cells into mitosis, fix a lesion in DNA, and, thus, increase the incidence of leukemia or shorten the latency between exposure and ultimate development of leukemia.

LD$_{50}$ Single Dose of Uniform Penetrating Radiation

The mortality response of humans to total-body uniform radiation is not known precisely. Cronkite and Bond[18] approached the problem by looking at the Marshallese response to 1.75 Gy total-body radiation and the response of animals in general. It appears that the near-maximal sublethal dose of radiation is about 2 Gy. By using the slope of many mammalian dose mortality curves, one can estimate that about 2.25 Gy would produce 5-percent to 10-percent mortality, and about 5 Gy would produce 90-percent mortality. The LD$_{50}$ would be approximately 3.6 Gy in the absence of treatment. It is established that the LD$_{50}$ is increased by the use of antibiotics to control infections, platelet transfusions to control bleeding, and (it is now clear) hematopoietic molecular regulators to stimulate early recovery of hematopoiesis.

Inadequacy of Physical Dose Estimates for Predicting Survival

In laboratory studies on animals or therapeutic exposure of patients, radiation exposure is deliberately designed for maximum uniformity of deposited energy in all tissues. In this situation, the dose in tissue is meaningful and useful. The exposure geometry is designed to minimize the effects of inverse square, attenuation, and scatter of impinging photons. The photons hit electrons and are accelerated in tissue at energies from near that of the impinging photon to near zero. With doses exceeding several cGy, the number of Compton electrons hitting the reference nuclear volume of 270×10^{-12} cm is large and uniform. As doses fall below 1 cGy, the number of electrons absorbed in a reference nucleus approaches 1, and, with lower doses, the fraction of cells hit decreases. The average absorbed dose per hit cell becomes a constant, with number of cells hit progressively decreasing as the dose decreases. This is important in considering the risk of carcinogenesis from small doses of radiation. The cells at risk receive a constant dose with fewer cells involved. Thus, there is a point at which the average calculated tissue dose from internal or external radiation becomes totally meaningless with low-level exposure.

The distribution of dose in tissue-equivalent phantoms for different point sources[19] is illustrated in figure 1. The sources are 250-kVp x ray, cobalt-60, 2,000-kVp x ray, and initial bomb gamma radiation. The widely different patterns of energy deposition are evident. For the 250-kVp x ray, there is a large buildup of energy deposition in the first 2-3 cm, followed by a decrease, as the result of inverse square and attenuation. Hematopoietic stem cells (HSC) located in the first 2-3 cm receive a much higher dose than the HSC in the exit 2-3 cm. For such a situation there is no single dose that can be used for prediction. In fact, single dose is less important than distribution of dose to HSC and the effect that these doses have upon the clonal survival of HSC—the time

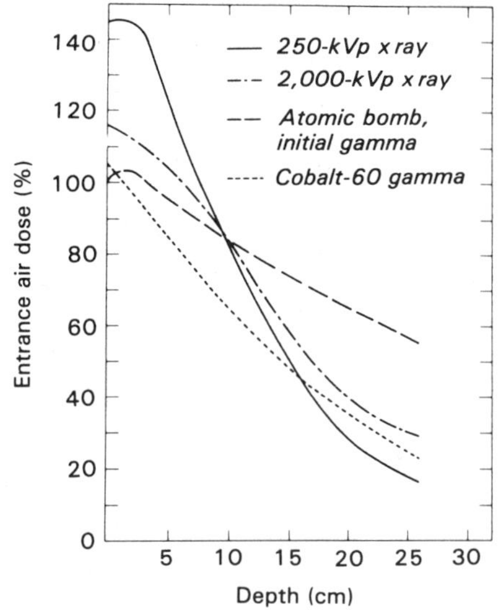

Figure 1. Phantom depth dose curves for different unilateral sources of radiation. The 250-kVp x ray, 2,000-kVp x ray, and cobalt-60 are essentially point sources with substantial inverse square effects. Atomic bomb gamma radiation is a broad source delivered at a distance in which the inverse square effects are negligible.

that these cells must rest before responding to molecular factors that control their self-renewal and differentiation.

In figure 2, depth-dose curves in a tissue-equivalent phantom are shown for initial bomb gamma radiation and mixed wide spectrum beta-gamma radiation.[17] An air dose or surface dose with fallout radiation may be over 10 Gy, but the meaningful tissue dose would be sublethal, about 1 Gy. An air dose of 1 Gy from initial bomb gamma radiation would represent the dose to the first 3-4 cm of tissue on the proximal side; the tissue dose to the distal 2-3 cm would be 50-60 percent of the dose to the proximal side. There is, then, a radiation dose in air at which the HSC near the proximal surface will be killed, and some HSC near the distal surface will survive and rescue the casualty.

Figure 3 shows the effect of exposure geometry and energy on mortality from the studies of Tullis et al.[20] on irradiation of swine by unilateral, bilateral, and atomic bomb gamma radiation. The LD$_{50}$ for unilateral 200-kVp x ray is 5 Gy in air. For bilateral radiation, the LD$_{50}$ is 4 Gy, and 2.3 Gy for atomic bomb gamma radiation.[21]

In radiation accidents, the heterogeneity of absorbed dose in tissue is even more marked. Hands and feet may receive many Gy, with ultimate destruction of tissue necessitating amputation. More distant bone marrow may receive only a few Gy or less with a lifesaving number of HSC surviving. These HSC,

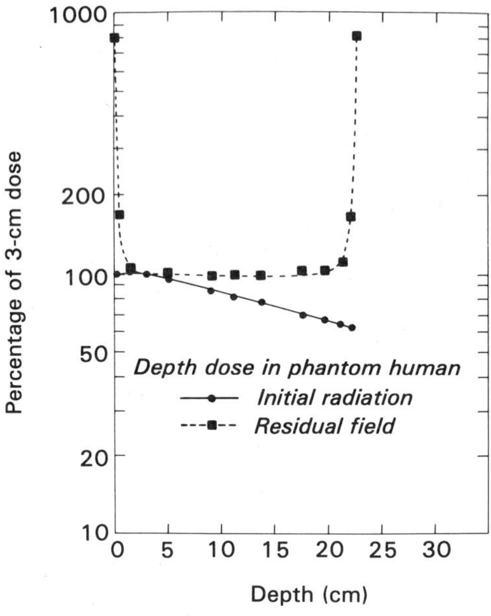

Figure 2. Comparison of depth dose curves for deposition of energy in tissue-equivalent phantoms for initial gamma radiation from an atomic bomb and from a fallout field of fission products from an atomic bomb. The dose in tissue is expressed as a percentage of the 3-cm dose in tissue, because air and surface dose from beta and low gamma radiation is high, with little penetrating power.

given time, will self-renew and differentiate into the different hematopoietic lineages restoring hematopoiesis. A radiation dosimeter worn close to the feet or hands would show a fatal dose of radiation. A dosimeter further away, however, on the side away from radiation, would record a lesser dosage to hands or feet and correctly predict a reasonable probability of survival. Thus, single personnel dosimeters will rarely be helpful in accidents.[22] Painstaking reconstruction of the accident, involving movement of exposed personnel and estimation of dose, is required to approximate the variation of absorbed dose to critical organ systems, such as intestine and bone marrow. This requires a mock-up, when possible, to measure dose rate at various positions in air and the conversion to absorbed dose distribution in tissue, a time-consuming procedure. Clinical decisions are required and must be made on the basis of signs and symptoms, not on the basis of air dose.

The physician's desire for a radiation dose and its probable mortality is understandable. If estimated mortality rate is approaching 100 percent, management will be more aggressive, using all available therapeutic armamentaria. If estimated mortality is low, watchful waiting is justified. In the case of accidental poisoning, the agent is known, but the dose is usually very uncertain. The therapy is determined by the properties of the agent and the clinical signs and symptoms, as with radiation accidents.

The doses of radiation estimated in recent radiation accidents were not for the most part physically measured or calculated doses based on source strength.

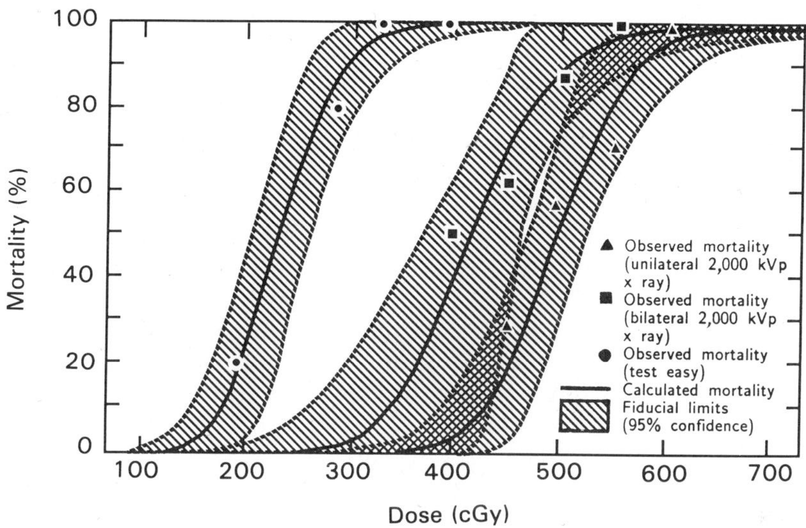

Figure 3. Dose mortality curves for swine for unilateral and bilateral 2,000-kVp x ray and for initial atomic bomb gamma radiation. The 2,000-kVp x ray produces a substantial inverse square effect. But the gamma radiation produces a negligible inverse square effect, because the bomb source is a broad beam delivered from a distance. (Previously published in *Radiology*, Volume 62, 1954.)

The doses are derived from biological response—chromosomal aberrations and lymphocyte, granulocyte, and platelet counts. Such doses are not a measured physical entity. Markedly different doses in air will produce equivalent depression in total lymphocyte, granulocyte, and platelet counts. The determinant of survival probability is the number of HSC that survive and the time they require to undergo self-renewal and differentiation into the lifesaving hematopoietic lineages.

The importance of surviving HSC is demonstrated by several experimental studies. Swift et al.[23] delivered a fatal dose of radiation to half of the body of rats and as quickly as possible moved the lead shield to the irradiated half and delivered a fatal dose to the shielded half. In that short interval migratory HSC had migrated into the shielded area in sufficient numbers to provide protection. Brecher and Cronkite[4] fatally irradiated one parabiotic rat while the other was shielded. HSC or other cells migrated from the shielded parabiont in sufficient number to protect it from fatal irradiation. Shielding of a mouse's leg (about 6 percent of bone marrow) or spleen provides marked protection from otherwise fatal irradiation to the rest of the body.

A physically derived or measured dose in Gy or a biologically derived dose, except under rigidly controlled conditions in the laboratory, is of limited, if any, value. Accident casualties have a markedly heterogeneous deposition of radiation energy that may result in late necrosis of proximal tissue and survival of HSC in distal tissues. The methodology developed by Fliedner *et al.*,[13] which predicts survival of HSC based on sequence of events involving changes in blood lymphocytes, granulocytes, and platelets, appears to be the most clinically useful approach to predict survival and guide therapy.

Combined Injuries

The management of burns and trauma takes precedence over radiation injury. The mortality of radiation injury is clearly increased by concomitant trauma and thermal injuries. Surgery should be completed before granulocytopenia and thrombocytopenia develop.

Conclusion

There are no mysteries about pathogenesis of the radiation syndromes. Common clinical sense directs management. A few areas in which further research is desirable are the following:

- Search for molecular regulators controlling growth of the GI epithelium and their application controlling the GI syndrome.
- Application of single and multiple hematopoietic molecular regulators in (1) accelerating host marrow and/or transplanted bone marrow regeneration and (2) determining if the use of these regulators will increase the incidence of hematopoietic or solid neoplasms or shorten the latency between irradiation and appearance of tumors.
- Analysis of hematological data on humans to predict the probability of survival and to provide a guide for appropriate supportive and replacement therapy.

Acknowledgment

Research was supported by U.S. Department of Energy contract DE-AC02-76CH00016.

References

1. Chiari, O. M. Preliminary communication on bone marrow transplantation. *Munch Med Wochenschr* 59:2503, 1912.
2. Fabricius-Moller, J. *Experimental Studies on the Hemorrhagic Diathesis of X-ray Sickness*. Levin and Munksgards, Forlag, Copenhagen, 1922.
3. Jacobson, L. O., Simmons, E. L., Marks, E. K., *et al.* Recovery from radiation injuries. *Science* 113:510-511, 1951.

4. Brecher, G., and Cronkite, E. P. Post-radiation parabiosis and survival in rats. *Proc Soc Exp Biol Med* 77:292-294, 1951.
5. Lorenz, E., Congdon, C., and Uphoff, D. Modification of acute irradiation injury in mice and guinea pigs. *Radiology* 58:863-877, 1952.
6. Ford, C. E., Lamerton, J. L., Barns, D. W. H., *et al.* Cytological identification of radiation chimaeras. *Nature* 177:452-454, 1956.
7. Bond, V. P., Cronkite, E. P., and Conard, R. A. Acute whole body radiation injury: Pathogenesis, pre- and post-radiation protection. In: *Atomic Medicine.* 5th Edition. C. F. Behrens, Ed. Williams and Wilkins Co., Baltimore, 1969, pp. 189-220.
8. Cronkite, E. P., Bond, V. P., and Conard, R. A. The hematology of ionizing radiation. In: *Atomic Medicine.* 5th edition. C. F. Behrens, Ed. Williams and Wilkins Co., Baltimore, 1969, pp. 221-261.
9. Oughtersen, A. W., and Warren, S. *Medical Effects of the Atomic Bomb in Japan.* McGraw-Hill Book Co., New York, 1956.
10. Hubner, K. F., and Fry, S. A., Eds. *The Medical Basis for Radiation Accident Preparedness.* Elsevier North Holland, Inc., New York, 1980.
11. Brecher, G., Cronkite, E. P., Conard, R. A., *et al.* Gastric lesion in experimental animal following single exposure to ionizing radiation. *Am J Pathol* 34:105-119, 1958.
12. Jacobs, G. J., Lynch, F. X., Cronkite, E. P., *et al.* Human radiation injury: A correlation of leukocyte depression with mortality in the Japanese exposed to the atomic bombs. *Milit Med* 128:732-739, 1963.
13. Fliedner, T. M., Steinbach, K. H., and Szepesi, T. Hematological indicators in the determination of clinical management strategies in radiation accidents. In: *Radiation Biological Effects Modifiers and Treatment.* Z. Qing-Xi and W. De-Chang, Eds. Chinese Medical Association, Beijing, China, 1988, pp. 60-91.
14. Cronkite, E. P. The diagnosis, prognosis and treatment of radiation injury produced by atomic bombs. *Radiology* 56:661-669, 1957.
15. Kikuchi, T., and Wakisaka, G. Hematological investigations of the atomic bomb sufferers in Hiroshima and Nagasaki cities. *Acta Sch Med Univ Kioto* 30:1-33, 1952.
16. Storb, R., Raff, R. F., Appelbaum, F. R., *et al.* What radiation dose for DLA-identical canine marrow grafts? *Blood* 72:1300-1304, 1988.
17. Cronkite, E. P., Bond, V. P., and Dunham, C. L. *Some Effects of Ionizing Radiation on Human Beings.* TID 5358. U.S. Atomic Energy Commission, Washington, DC, 1956 (U.S. Government Printing Office, Washington, DC).
18. Cronkite, E. P., and Bond, V. P. Diagnosis of radiation injury and analysis of the human lethal dose of radiation. *U.S. Armed Forces Medical Journal* 11:249-260, 1960.
19. Bond, V. P., Cronkite, E. P., Sondhaus, C. A., *et al.* Influence of exposure geometry on the pattern of radiation dose delivered to large animal phantoms. *Radiat Res* 6:554-572, 1957.
20. Tullis, J. L., Chambers, F. W., Morgan, J. E., *et al.* Mortality in swine and dose distribution studies in phantoms exposed to supervoltage radiation. *Am J Roentgenol* 67:620-627, 1952.
21. Tullis, J. L., Lamson, B. G., and Madden, S. G. Mortality in swine exposed to gamma radiation from an atomic bomb source. *Radiology* 62:409-415, 1954.
22. National Council on Radiation Protection and Measurements. *Radiological Factors Affecting Decision-Making in a Nuclear Attack.* NCRP Report 42. Washington, DC, 1974.
23. Swift, M. N., Taketa, S. T., and Bond, V. P. Regionally fractionated x-irradiation equivalent in dose to total-body exposure. *Radiat Res* 1:241-252, 1954.

Acute Effects of Radiation Exposure Following the Chernobyl Accident

Immediate Results of Radiation Sickness and Outcome of Treatment

Angelina K. Guskova, N. M. Nadezhina,
Anjelika V. Barabanova, Alexandr E. Baranov,
I. A. Gusev, Tatiana G. Protasova,
V. B. Boguslavskij, and V. N. Pokrovskaya

Information on the conditions of irradiation and clinical records of the acute radiation sickness (ARS) in victims of the accident at the Chernobyl nuclear power plant were reported in August 1986.[1,2] Prognostic evaluations of the outcomes of the hematopoietic injuries were presented in April 1987.[3] Data on the early effects of the radiation were also included in an appendix to the United Nations Scientific Committee on the Effects of Atomic Radiation (UNSCEAR) Report.[4] Further in-depth analysis of the clinical phase of ARS has been ongoing. Some results of this analysis are presented in this chapter.

Earlier opinion about the relative significance of the separate components of combined injury were fully confirmed by the clinical, anatomical, laboratory, and cardiological analyses and by the pathological (anatomical) and biophysical postmortem investigations.[1,2] Except for two patients (24 and 25) who had ARS and thermal burns, all others were primarily affected by total-body uniform beta-gamma irradiation. The action of penetrating radiation on the total body was the primary reason for development of the clinical syndromes of ARS (such as bone marrow and gastrointestinal syndromes and their combinations), which are characteristic for a dose range of 1-16 Gy. Beta radiation, penetrating only to the depth of skin (T. G. Protsova and T. I. Davydovskaya, personal communication), at doses at least 10-20 times higher than the average total-body dose was the cause of the vast radiation injuries to the skin in more than half of the patients. These injuries significantly complicated the clinical course of ARS and influenced the outcome. Isolated centers of deeper local radiation injuries appeared on shallow radiation injuries as a result of contact

A. K. GUSKOVA, A. E. BARANOV, T. G. PROTASOVA, Biophysical Institute of the U.S.S.R. Ministry of Health, Moscow 123182, Jhivopisnaia 46, U.S.S.R., and Clinical Hospital 6, Moscow, U.S.S.R.; A. V. BARABANOVA, International Atomic Energy Agency, Vienna, Austria; N. M. NADEZHINA, I. A. GUSEV, V. B. BOGUSLAVSKIJ, V. N. POKROVSKAYA, All-Union Institute of Technical and Scientific Information, Academy of Science, Moscow, U.S.S.R.

Treatment of Radiation Injuries, Edited by
D. Browne *et al.,* Plenum Press, New York, 1990

                                                        A. K. Guskova et al.

with objects that were contaminated by radionuclides, such as wet clothes or boots.

No correlation was found between the radionuclide content measured during clinical manifestations and postmortem investigations. Radionuclide incorporation did not contribute to the clinical picture of the ARS prodromal phase for a given radiation dose. Radionuclide incorporation was measured by gamma spectrometric measurements of blood samples (I. A. Gusev and A. A. Moiseev, personal communication), urine (R. D. Drutman and V. V. Mordasheva, personal communication), and postmortem samples of organs and tissues (I. A. Gusev and V. I. Popov, personal communication). Maximal amounts of activity were as follows: patient 24, 5 mCi iodine-131, 2 mCi cesium-137, and 2 mCi cesium-134; patient 25, 1 mCi iodine-131, 2.5 mCi cesium-137, and 2 mCi cesium-134. Contamination by cerium-144 was not higher than 30 μCi, with about 95 percent of cerium activity deposited in the lungs. Other radionuclide content (for example, zirconium-95, niobium-95, ruthenium-103, ruthenium-106, lanthanum-140, barium-140, cerium-141) was not higher than maximal permissible intakes for each radionuclide separately.

Although the paths of intake in patients 24 and 25 (through the damaged skin or by inhalation) are not quite clear, the doses of internal irradiation at times of death (conservatively evaluated) for patient 24 were 30 Gy for the thyroid gland, 2 Gy for the total body, and 2.5 Gy for the lungs. For patient 25, the doses were 6 Gy for the thyroid gland, 1 Gy for the total body, and 2 Gy for the lungs.

For personnel who were at the plant at the time of the accident, the mean dose of irradiation in the lungs from internal emitters was 20 cGy; in the thyroid, 250 cGy; and in the total body, about 15 cGy. Table 1 provides data on the internal irradiation of personnel who died as a result of irradiation.

The clinical characteristics of the main syndromes of ARS during the prodromal phase and syndrome combinations with each other and with local

Table 1. Internal Irradiation Doses of Expired Patients

Patient	Thyroid dose (Gy)	Lung dose (Gy)	Total-body dose (Gy)	
			Internal	External (gamma)
24	30.0	2.5	2.0	1.7
25	6.0	2.0	1.0	4.7
17	1.0	0.4	0.2	10.0
3	0.3	0.3	0.2	12.0
4	1.2	0.4	0.1	11.0
26	0.5	0.3	0.1	12.0

Data are only for patients with the highest internal doses. Doses are at time of death.

radiation injuries were presented in several reports.[1,2,5-7] Figure 1 shows the relationships and frequencies of lethal outcomes in the different groups of affected personnel. At third and fourth degree ARS, nearly all patients had severe bone marrow syndrome combined with skin and mucosal injuries. In 80 percent of the patients with fourth degree ARS, the gastrointestinal syndrome developed, and in 7 patients, pneumonitis with pronounced respiratory insufficiency was observed. The complication of pronounced and/or extensive skin injuries was evident in all patients. For those with radiation burns over more than 40 percent of body-surface area (two-thirds of the patients with expected lethal outcomes), burns should be considered, based on clinical data, as the leading cause of the outcome of ARS. Skin lesions were the cause of death in five patients. Skin injuries were significant for early as well as delayed times of death.

The manner of grouping patients according to the prognostic development of ARS at different stages of observation in order to choose the appropriate therapy has been given in detail in several publications.[6-9] In this chapter we discuss only the practical significance of such characteristics as the number of lymphocytes on the first 3-7 days after exposure, the number of neutrophils on days 7 and 8, the time period to reach a neutrophil count < 1,000 at 1-5 weeks of observation, and the period of development of pronounced thrombocytopenia (from 2 weeks until the end of the latent phase; for first degree ARS, 4-6 weeks from the time of exposure) (see figure 2). The highly significant data from the karyotype analysis of bone marrow lymphocytes and peripheral blood lymphocytes as well as the results of direct count of dividing cells in biopsy preparations of hematopoietic organs have been discussed earlier,[1,8] and have been confirmed later by quantitative indicators. The dynamics of the blood parameters provided the quantitative indicators for the subsequent course of ARS.

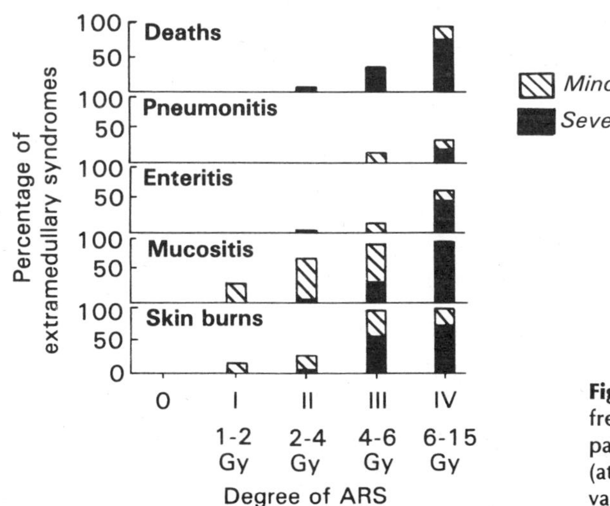

Figure 1. Extramedullary syndrome frequencies for various dose ranges of patients from the Chernobyl accident (at acute radiation sickness (ARS) of various degrees).

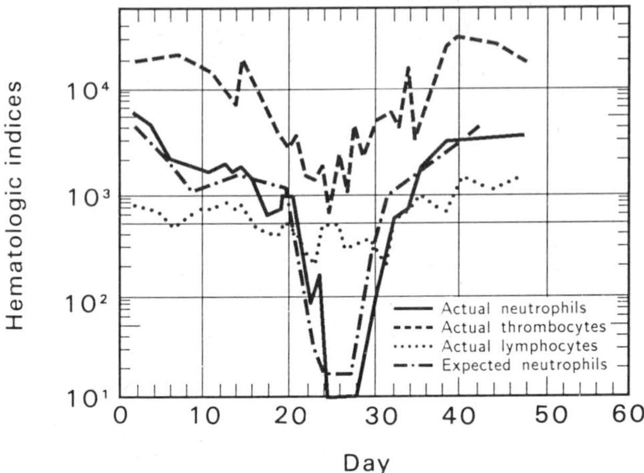

Figure 2. Expected and actual peripheral blood parameter in victims of the Chernobyl accident.

Other clinical (neurological and ophthalmological) and laboratory (immunological, coagulation, and metabolic) tests have mainly shown the correlation with separate clinical syndromes of ARS and its complications (nerve system injuries, toxemia, and bleeding). For biochemical tests (I. P. Turina, M. P. Tarakanova, and T. A. Ivanova, personal communication), the correlation with severity of ARS was best for some indicators of protein metabolism and enzymatic activity.[1,7] Pronounced hypoalbuminemia from 1 day to 30 days after exposure was observed in patients with severe degrees of ARS (especially with gastrointestinal injuries) and large surface areas of beta-dermatitis (figure 3).

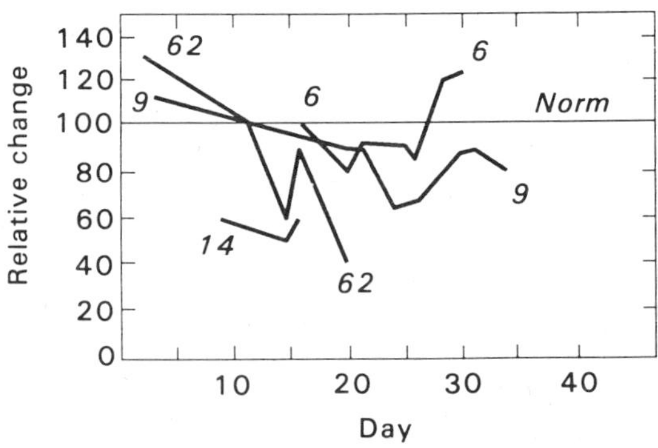

Figure 3. Albumin content in blood serum of patients from the Chernobyl accident with third or fourth degree acute radiation sickness (ARS). Injured skin surface area and degree of radiation injury: patient 14, 60 percent, third and fourth degree ARS; patient 62, 90 percent, second and third degree ARS; patient 6, 50 percent, second and third degree ARS; patient 9, 46 percent, first and second degree ARS.

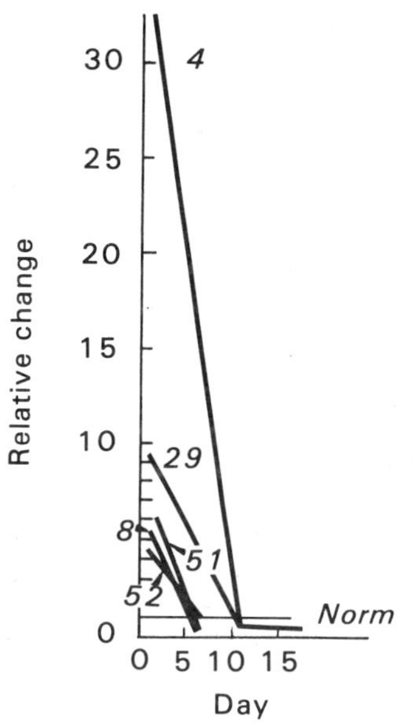

Figure 4. Activity of blood serum α-amylase in patients from the Chernobyl accident with various degrees of acute radiation sickness (ARS). Degrees of ARS and oropharyngeal syndrome (OPS): patients 4, 29, and 8, fourth degree ARS and fourth degree OPS; patient 51, second degree ARS and first degree OPS; patient 52, third degree ARS and second degree OPS.

In the critical phase of ARS, the maximal manifestations of infection and inflammatory and necrotic changes coincided with periods of increases in α_1 and α_2 globulins. The increase in α-amylase activity at 1-5 days correlated with the severity of general manifestation of ARS and especially with subsequent oropharyngeal syndrome (figure 4). The increase in activity of creatine kinase at 3-10 days correlated with the size of injured skin surface area and severity of beta dermatitis (figure 5; table 2). In the critical phase of ARS and in cases of complications, increased enzyme activity was observed as a small second wave of increased activity of creatine-phosphokinase and as an increase in blood alanine aminotransferase, asparaginotransferase, and gamma glutamine transpeptidase (figure 6). An increase in creatinine and urea in the blood (and urine) was noted in the terminal phase of extremely sick patients (figure 7). However, the changes in all these indicators rarely reached extreme values because of corrective therapy. These indicators clearly showed positive dynamics in all patients who survived. In the patients who died, the fatal character of indicator changes appeared only in the last days of their lives. Bone marrow transplantation complicated by secondary illness[3,5] was reflected in the dynamics of biochemical indicators that were used particularly for identification of secondary illness.

An analysis was also made of neuroimmunological changes in comparison with the clinical neurological picture. These changes included titers of circulating antibodies to brain antigen and myelin protein, reaction of inhibition of migration and specific agglomeration of leukocytes, and quantitative

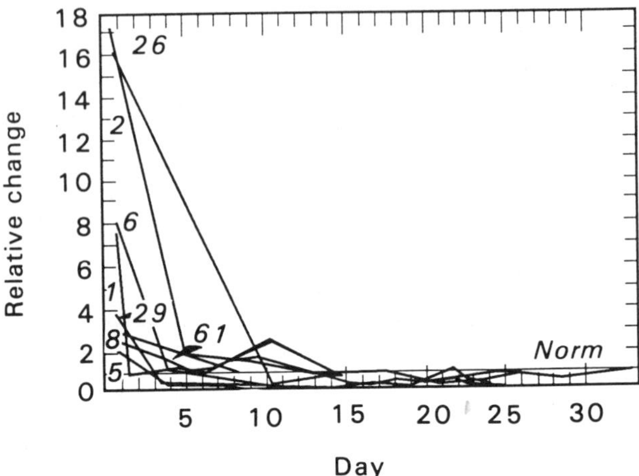

Figure 5. Activity of creatine kinase in patients from the Chernobyl accident.

relationship of T and B lymphocytes in accelerated reaction of rosette formation (I. N. Shakirova and L. I. Muravieva, personal communication). The analysis showed that, after general irradiation, the threshold value of the dose after which minimal signs of microdestruction of brain tissue could be found by immunological tests during the prodromal phase of ARS is about 2 Gy. The intensity of neuroimmunological shifts was a result of toxic influences of local radiation injuries. In the course of these studies, a computer program for the

Table 2. Degree of Skin Radiation Injury, Size of Injured Skin Surface, and Degree of Acute Radiation Sickness in Patients From the Chernobyl Accident

Patient	Degree of skin radiation injury[1]	Injured skin (percent)	Degree of ARS radiation sickness[2]
1	2°, 3°	50	IV
2	2°, 3°	96	IV
5	2°	6	III
6	1°, 2°, 3°	46	IV
8	1°, 2°	25	IV
26	2°, 3°	60	IV
29	1°, 2°, 3°	40	IV
61	1°, 2°	18	II

[1]Degrees of skin radiation injury: 1°, mild; 2°, moderate; 3°, severe.
[2]Degrees of acute radiation sickness: I, mild; II, moderate; III, severe; IV, lethal.

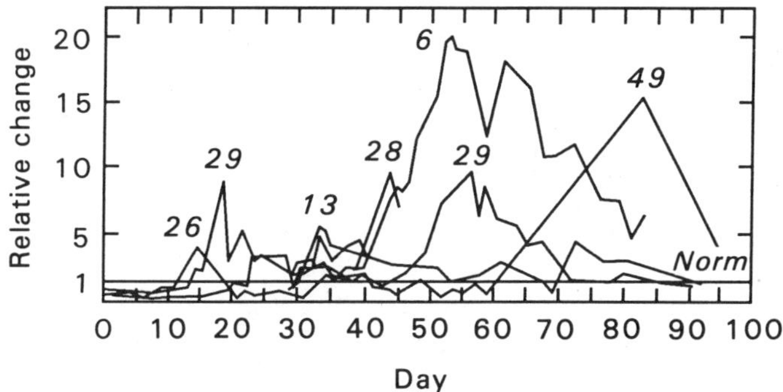

Figure 6. Activity of alanine aminotransferase in patients from the Chernobyl accident at various test periods. Degrees of acute radiation sickness (ARS): patient 49, second degree ARS; patient 13, third degree ARS; patients 6, 26, 28, 29, fourth degree ARS.

use of the data of coded sickness histories of neurological syndrome was created and tested (I. N. Shakirova and S. M. Shendyapin, personal communication).

The state of hemostasis in the accident victims was determined by direct action of ionizing radiation (thrombocytopoiesis, structural changes of blood vessel walls) as well as indirect action (L. S. Pochukaeva, personal communication). Activation of the coagulation pathway during the prodromal phase of ARS was found (increase in maximal activity of thrombin and thromboplastin in autocoagulation test, and permanent presence in the patient's blood of soluble fibrin monomeric complexes). These changes could promote

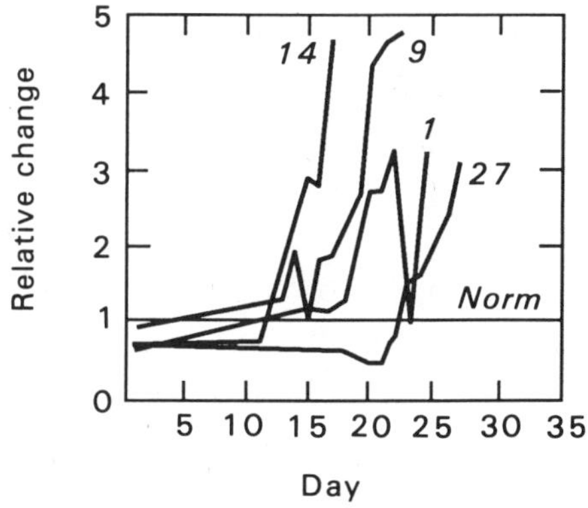

Figure 7. Characteristic changes in serum urea of patients from the Chernobyl accident. Degrees of acute radiation sickness (ARS): patient 27, third degree ARS; patients 1, 9, and 14, fourth degree ARS.

intravascular coagulation of blood. The increase in fibrinolysis during the latent phase of ARS of intermediate degree could result in dissolution of fibrin complexes. In especially severe cases of injury, this mechanism of feedback was lacking, and the blockage of fibrinolysis led to precipitation of fibrin and formation of blood clots in microcirculatory vessels; blockage could have led to the disruption of organ function and to the secondary changes of the vessel walls. With the activation of hemostasis and the presence of microclots and microthrombi, there was an enhanced inclination for hemorrhage even in the injuries of minor vessels. Thus, the reaction was paradoxical—hemostasis activation was not leading to hemostatic effect (figure 8).

After observing patients for 18 months, no need arose to reconsider the criteria of diagnosis of second, third, and fourth degree ARS. The course of ARS in the prodromal phase as well as in the recovery phase corresponded to our previous data about peculiarities of ARS resulting from total-body,

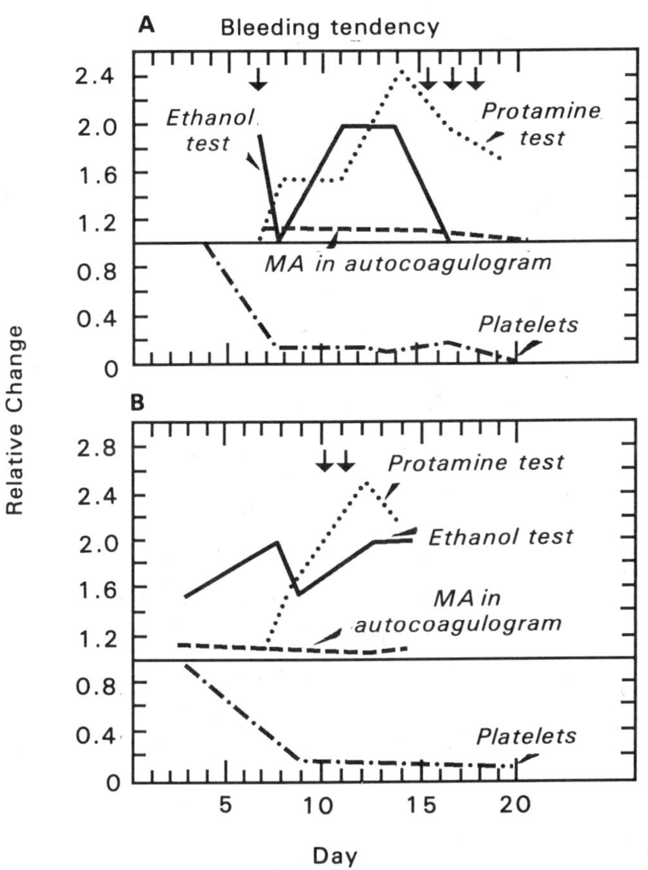

Figure 8. Characteristic ratios of hemostasis indices in patients from the Chernobyl accident with acute radiation sickness (ARS) and deep venous thrombosis. Arrows mark the manifestations of bleeding tendency. Patient 26 (A) and patient 25 (B) received plasma and heparin therapy.

relatively uniform exposure to the indicated dose ranges.[8,9] It seemed appropriate to go back and give special attention to the criteria of diagnosis of slight degrees of ARS and to the few observations in the subclinical dose to document more distinctly at what dose levels and in what time frame the individually significant clinical signs of the reaction to exposure were revealed.[8-10]

Careful analysis of complete blood counts and observations made in specialized inpatient facilities revealed that regular changes in leukocyte and platelet counts appeared only at 5-6 weeks after exposure. There may have been a shift of these symptoms for several days (about 1 week), with an earlier change in platelet count. The primary reaction could be seen in different degrees, but appeared regularly in the later stages (up to several hours after irradiation) and only in such signs as nausea and vomiting. The external exposure doses in this group of patients, according to the data from cytogenetic analysis (frequency of dicentrics), were in the range of 0.8-2 Sv (80-200 rem).

Considering the cytogenetic data for persons who in the early stages of observation were thought to have first degree ARS because of the above-mentioned and other symptoms, the following regularities were found (A. V. Barabanova, A. V. Sevankaev, and M. V. Konchalovskij, personal communication):

- Of 21 patients whose irradiation doses were estimated between 0 cGy and 60 cGy according to cytogenetic data, none showed the characteristic symptoms of ARS.
- In 20 patients with doses estimated according to cytogenetic data between 70 cGy and 210 cGy, it was possible to diagnose first degree ARS, and the dynamics of the neutrophil count indicated the mean doses in bone marrow to be about 100-200 cGy. Thus, a 70-cGy dose of total-body irradiation could be tentatively considered a minimal dose, leading to weakness and regular significant changes in the blood that are characteristic of first degree ARS.
- The cytogenetic data and the whole dynamics of neutrophil counts retrospectively validate the diagnosis of first degree ARS. The diagnosis is possible for irradiated persons even in the absence of information on dose levels, as well as when some information about borderline doses (60-120 cGy) is present.

We used these criteria systematically with the available methods of dose reconstruction to illustrate the characteristic dynamics of neutrophil counts in first degree ARS (figure 9). The first variant of the diagnostic computer program unifying the diagnostic approaches to first degree ARS was developed. The assessment of effectiveness of treatment was also analyzed. Principles and direct results of treatment of ARS for different degrees of severity were discussed in several reports.[6,7]

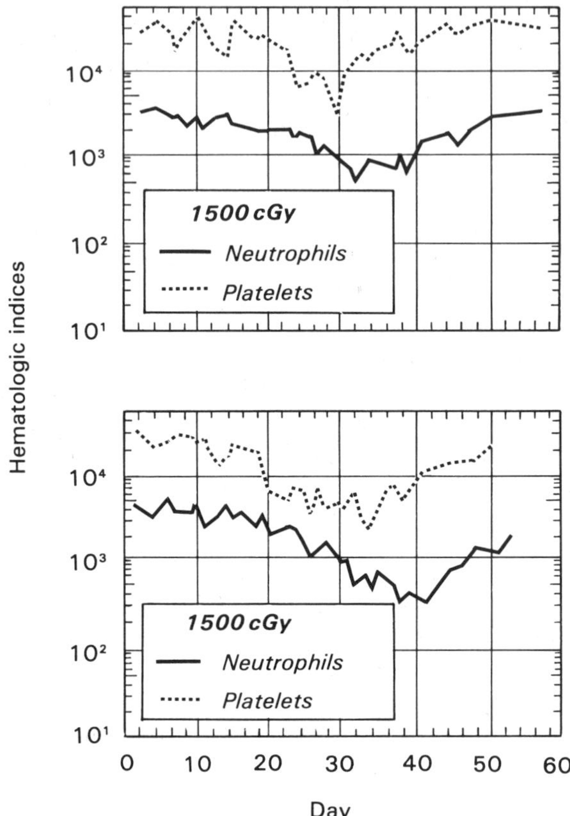

Figure 9. Characteristic curves of leukocyte (neutrophils) and platelet counts in two patients with minor degree acute radiation sickness.

The analysis of the causes of lethal outcomes and the data on the dynamics of clinical and laboratory indicators of living patients studied to date serve as additional criteria on the effectiveness of treatment. Preliminary results of these two aspects of observations follow.

As stated before, 28 patients with third or fourth degree ARS died, and 1 patient with second degree ARS died. Two of these patients had combined thermoradiation injuries. The times of death varied from 11 days to 96 days. The data from the principal elements of the pathological picture of the patients are given. Especially emphasized are the cases with unusual causes of death for a given time of observation.

For all patients the pronounced severity of the course of sickness was due to combinations of two to three clinical syndromes and complex spectrums of toxic and infectious complications and circulatory deficiencies. The skin lesions covering significant parts of body surface were a leading cause of death for all stages from the time of irradiation. For deaths occurring earlier than day 24, the skin lesions were accompanied not only with severe disruption of hematopoiesis but also with early pronounced gastrointestinal syndrome. As life expectancy increased, the skin injuries were more frequently connected with one or two syndromes of ARS or acquired independent significance in the outcome of the sickness.

The combinations of syndromes, their complications, and the direct causes of death were more varied from 24 days to 48 days after exposure. By excluding some of these complicating circumstances for the levels of ARS, it might have been possible to change the outcome of the sickness. In several patients with severe hematopoietic injury there were slight but distinct signs of a center of regeneration of bone marrow and of regenerating parts of intestinal mucosa. At the end of the second month, the extremely high severity of infectious (including viral) complications was typical, as dystrophic changes in parenchymal organs were also. For many patients and for different stages, the various circulatory dysfunctions in capillaries were characteristically localized most frequently to the lungs, gastrointestinal tract, and in the brain. However, heavy, fatal hemorrhages were rare.

In general, the complex treatment measures for ARS were quite effective.[1,2] The analysis of the effect of bone marrow transplantation for the limited group of patients has been published previously.[5,11]

It is difficult to assess other components of this treatment. However, on the basis of postmortem morphological studies, it is possible to discuss the definite effectiveness of the prophylactic system of therapy of infections, especially bacterial infections. Control of infections was achieved by isolating patients, organizing special aseptic regimens for the patients during the period of agranulocytosis, therapeutic and prophylactic use of antimicrobial and antifungal drugs, and in some cases, local application or injection of an antiviral drug (acyclovir). The diagnosis of sepsis (in 4 cases, mixed fungal and bacterial, and, in 3 cases, bacterial) was confirmed after pathological and postmortem microbiological studies only in 7 of 28 persons who died of third or fourth degree ARS. In others, microbial contamination of tissues was not pronounced, and only an insignificant number of bacterial colonies was noted from necrotic surfaces of skin and mucosa.

The other important component of the treatment regimen was the blood component replacement therapy. The direct effectiveness of allogeneic and autologous, cryopreserved platelets (thrombocytes) should be especially stressed. For a patient with second degree ARS or third degree ARS, three to eight transfusions of platelets (3×10^{11}/treatment) were used on the average. The regimen ensured the absence of life-threatening bleeding for the overwhelming majority of patients with the bone marrow syndrome of ARS that was not aggravated by other syndromes. This effect was observed even in long-term (14-20 days) and profound ($<$ 5,000 cells/μL) thrombocytopenia.

As the direct cause of death, the hemorrhagic complication was observed in only one patient. In this case, hemorrhage was provoked by traumatic manipulation when a catheter was inserted in the subclavicular vein.

Total parenteral nutrition was given for the correction of metabolic disturbances and in cases of possible direct gastrointestinal mucosa insult. All necessary means for symptomatic therapy were also used in cases of signs of brain edema, nephrotoxicity, hepatotoxicity, and circulatory and hypoxic encephalopathy. However, the combination of two or three syndromes as a rule was fatal.

Because of these facts it is hardly possible to estimate the LD_{50} as mentioned at the experts meeting in August 1986.[1] A general qualitative characteristic of therapeutic effectiveness could be the frequency of lethal outcomes for groups of patients with different degrees of ARS.

As mentioned above, only 1 of 55 patients with second degree ARS, whose irradiation dose was 210 cGy, died of ARS. Of 21 patients with third degree ARS (dose range between 400 cGy and 600 cGy), 14 survived. All patients except one with fourth degree ARS died. As the analysis of pathological data shows, the deaths came as a result of combinations of several clinical syndromes, primarily the combination of gastrointestinal and bone marrow syndromes with total or subtotal skin injuries. The times of death after combined thermoradiation injuries were 16 days and 23 days in the presence of a slight degree of gastrointestinal injury for one patient and of bone marrow injury for the other. This shows the significant contributing role of skin injury to the deaths of patients 25 and 24. Breathing problems were of complex, nonuniform nature for patients who died at various times. According to pathological studies, breathing problems were significantly pronounced for 13 patients and were especially significant for 7 of those 13. There were signs of expressed circulatory disturbances in the injuries at the alveolar-capillary level, interstitial edema for all periods of observation, and typical fibrillar-hemorrhagic manifestations in patients who died at later times. The dynamic observations of all patients with ARS were continued for 18 months to assess completeness of recovery. During hematopoietic recovery, the blood parameters were restored to normal in 84 percent of patients after 12-18 months.

We found that patients recovered completely during the prodromal phase, even of severe ARS (V. N. Pokrovskaya and N. M. Nadezhina, personal communication). Moderate, not very stable leukopenia and more rarely thrombocytopenia were manifested in the latest observations of 9 percent, 15 percent, and 30 percent of patients who had first degree, second degree, and third degree ARS, respectively. At the same time, in 50 percent of patients with incomplete recovery even at the first observation, a moderate decrease in the number of leukocytes and/or platelets was noted, indicating insufficient hematopoiesis. At later times, the moderate unstable cytopenia evidently increased due to the gastrointestinal injury of ARS (hepatitis, gastritis, ulcer). All patients with third degree ARS suffered from local radiation injuries. For those with prolonged cytopenia, treatment that included plastic surgery was necessary.

The studies on the capacity to perform physical work and of energy expenditures have shown favorable results for these indicators, which gradually increased during recovery from ARS (V. V. Charitonov and O. P. Efremovtseva, personal communication). The time and completeness of recovery depended to a certain degree on the severity of ARS or the irradiation dose. The group of patients without clinical signs of ARS in all periods of observation (up to 1 year) preserved the ability to work at significant levels of energy expenditure. Energy expenditures of 4.9 kcal/minute were characteristic for patients with first degree ARS. The patients with second and third degree ARS differed considerably from the previous groups of patients even during the latent phase of ARS; their ability to work was limited to energy expenditures not higher than 3.0-3.8 kcal/minute. For patients with first and second degree ARS the levels of physical ability were restored (already) at 8 weeks and 9 weeks, respectively; these levels remained high at the end of the year after irradiation. For patients with third degree ARS the indicators of capacity for work at the early phase of recovery were worse than initially (3.5 to 3.8 kcal/minute, respectively) and even by the end of the year had not reached normal levels. The reactions of individual patients to physical stress differed significantly because of differences in age, physical condition, and previous illnesses.

The results of clinical and psychological studies of neuropsychological activities are interesting (F. S. Torubarov, P. V. Chesalin, and O. V. Chinkina, personal communication). Complex stress and radiation situations resulted in moderate asthenia during the early recovery period (4-6 months after the accident) in some of the patients. Asthenic manifestations correlated in frequency and expressiveness with the severity of sickness (approximately 75 percent, 50 percent, and 35 percent in patients with third degree ARS, second degree ARS, and first degree ARS, respectively). However, the time to manifestation of asthenia correlated with the patient's premorbid peculiarities of personality, attitude to the risk of irradiation and ARS, degree of information, profession, future work, and normal life. Asthenia passed in 9-18 months, with recovery of the function of main organs and systems.

Our experience shows that, in choosing indicators or contraindicators for some kind of work, the multifactorial study of physical and psychological efficiency, self-estimation, psychic condition of personality, reactions, and peculiarities of personality for particular work have great practical significance. The choice of a working place and favorable social and personal rehabilitation help in recovering full capacity to work, even in patients who suffered second or third degree ARS.

Clinical and paraclinical methods of study indicate that the overwhelming majority of ARS patients (five of six patients) limit future contact with radiation sources. Only a small number of them, as a rule suffering from intercurrent illnesses, were limited in working regimens (for example, exclusion of night shifts, usage of protective cloth, gloves) (N. M. Nadezhina and A. V. Barabanova, personal communication). Residual manifestations of local radiation injuries, third degree ARS, or a combination of ARS with other illnesses temporarily disabled some patients for the next 1-2 years.

Dynamic observation of patients during the second year after the accident showed improvement in capacity for work in three of four of them, excluding three patients (one with local radiation injury and two with nonrational choice of working place). The possibility of gradually broadening their working and social activity exists. It should be noted, however, that a choice of work adequate to the general conditions of the person after ARS and a personal interest in this work favorably influence and stimulate functional recovery. Complete social and personal rehabilitation after ARS was clearly demonstrated to the whole world when our patient, L. P. Telatnikov, who now actively works at a center for training firemen, appeared on the television screens of Italy, Great Britain, and the United States. Such examples could be multiplied many times, including the cases when capacity for highly professional work was retained (with limited contact or without contact with radiation). These patients were engineers and operators of the Chernobyl nuclear power plant and suffered first or second degree ARS. Radiation doses of personnel working at the plant in 1987 were not higher than 0.6 rem.

References

1. USSR State Committee on the Utilization of Atomic Energy. The accident at Chernobyl nuclear power plant and its consequences. Information compiled for the Post-Accident Review Meeting, part II, Annex 7, Vienna, Austria, August 25-29, 1986.
2. International Nuclear Safety Advisory Group. Summary report on the post-accident review meeting on the Chernobyl accident. Vienna, Austria: International Atomic Energy Agency, 1986. (Safety Series No. 75-INSAG-1.)
3. Guskova, A. K., and Baranov, A. E. Hematologic effects in victims of Chernobyl NPP accident. Report for the Royal College of Pathologists, Low Levels of Radiation etc. Environmental Factors and Oncogenesis. United Kingdom, April 1987.
4. Guskova, A. K., Barabanova, A. V., Baranov, A. E., et al. Acute radiation effects in victims of the Chernobyl nuclear power plant accident. Appendix to *Sources Effects and Risks of Ionizing Radiation*, United Nations Scientific Committee on the Effects of Atomic Radiation. New York, 1988.
5. Baranov, A. E., et al. Bone marrow transplantation after whole-body irradiation in victims of the Chernobyl accident. *Ter Arkh* 1987.
6. Sevankaev, A. P. Radiosensitivity of chromosomes of human lymphocytes in mitotic cycle. *M Energoizdat*, 1987.

 7. Guskova, A. K. Acute effects in victims of the Chernobyl NPP accident. *Med Radiol (Mosk)* 12:3-18, 1987.
 8. Pyatkin, E. K., and Baranov, A. E. Biological indication of dose based on analysis of chromosome aberrations and numbers of cell in peripheral blood: Outcomes in science and technology. All-Union Institute of Technical and Scientific Information, Academy of Science, U.S.S.R. Ser *Radiat Biol* 3:103-179, 1980.
 9. Acute effects of irradiation in humans. GKAE SSSR, NKRZ pri Minzdrave SSSR, CNIatominform, 1986.
10. Guskova, A. K., and Shakirova, I. N. The main regularities of injuries action of radiation on human nervous system. Literature review. *Zh Nevropatol Psikhiatr*, 1988 (in press).
11. Baranov, A., Gale, R. P., Guskova, A., *et al*. Bone marrow transplantation after the Chernobyl nuclear accident. *N Engl J Med* 321(4):205-212, 1989.

Potential Role for Human Colony-Stimulating Factors in the Treatment of Radiation Injuries

William P. Peters

Introduction

Hematopoiesis in humans appears to be controlled by a series of growth factors that are responsible for accelerating the proliferation and lineage-specific differentiation of committed progenitors. More than 10 factors acting at different and overlapping steps of hematopoietic differentiation have now been identified, molecularly cloned, expressed *in vitro*, and, in some cases, evaluated in primates and in the clinical setting. Because it has been shown clinically that growth factors can enhance hematopoietic reconstitution in patients with severe bone marrow injury, these factors have potential for treating radiation injury. This review explores the biological and biochemical as well as the clinical aspects of the colony-stimulating factors (CSF's) currently in clinical use, particularly in relation to the treatment of nuclear accident injuries.

Biological and Biochemical Properties of Colony-Stimulating Factors

The CSF's act biologically to permit the survival of committed progenitors, to enhance their proliferation, to force differentiation, and, in many cases, to enhance or alter the function of mature effector cells that develop under the influence of the CSF. Some of these factors are constitutively expressed, and circulate in serum. The interregulation of the CSF's is incompletely understood. Regulation of the gene expression, as well as translation and secretion of completed products, is a complex, intricate system involving autocrine, paracrine, endocrine, and feedback mechanisms.

Several clinical products are currently being developed, including recombinant human granulocyte CSF (rhG-CSF), granulocyte-macrophage CSF

W. P. PETERS, Bone Marrow Transplant Program, Division of Hematology/Oncology, Department of Medicine, Duke University Medical Center, Durham, North Carolina 27701.

Treatment of Radiation Injuries, Edited by
D. Browne *et al.*, Plenum Press, New York, 1990

(rhGM-CSF), macrophage CSF (rhM-CSF, CSF-1), interleukin-1 (rhIL-1), interleukin-3 (rhIL-3), and erythropoietin. In some cases, both glycosylated and nonglycosylated variants of the molecule are being developed. Whether important differences in the biological activity, therapeutic efficacy, or toxicity are associated with these variances is yet uncertain. The protein products for GM-CSF lacking glycosylation appear, in general, to have a higher biological specific activity *in vitro*, although it is not clear that this will have important differences in clinical or toxic effects. Similarly, variations in products that are glycosylated using expression systems, such as yeast or the Chinese hamster ovary, may differ from the native glycosylated human product because they rely on nonhuman cell systems to produce the glycosylation on the molecule. In some settings, such as erythropoietin, glycosylation is extremely important to biological activity. The final importance of such differences in the biochemistry of these drugs will not be known until comparative clinical trials are undertaken.

Lineage Specificity

Although hematopoietic lineage specificity is implied in the names of G-CSF and GM-CSF, the implication may be misleading. *In vitro* evaluation has suggested that GM-CSF, for instance, has biological effects on lineages other than the granulocyte macrophage line, including burst-promoting activity and enhancement of megakaryocytic activity. Concern has been expressed about the detection of receptors for the human CSF's on the surface of nonhematopoietic cells. Although receptors for various hematopoietic growth factors can be identified on certain cell lines, particularly small-cell lung cancer, the biological importance of these receptors remains unclear. *In vitro* evaluations have demonstrated enhancement of proliferation, decrease of proliferation, and no effect on cell proliferation. In our studies, evaluation of various breast cancer cell lines has failed to produce evidence of significant neoplastic proliferation under the influence of rhGM-CSF or rhG-CSF.

Proliferation and Function

Although the CSF's have been identified predominantly because of their effects on inducing proliferation of certain committed bone marrow stem cells, these compounds also have been demonstrated to have significant effects on the functional capacity of mature effector cells. The effects on proliferation, differentiation, and functional aspects of mature effector cells are presented in table 1.

The effects on function are particularly diverse, and there are important differences among the CSF's that may have implications for their use in

Table 1. Comparative Effects of Myeloid Colony-Stimulating Factors[1]

Factor[2]	Proliferation[3]	Differentiation	Function[4]	Cascade Effects[5]
rhG-CSF	G-CFU GM-CFU M-CFU Small cell lung lines H-128 HL-60 KG-1 NSF-60	Human myeloid leukemia cells WEHI-3B myelomonocytic cells	Increases ADCC Enhances phagocytosis Enhances arachidonic acid release Enhances chemotaxis for granulocytes	Synergizes with IL-3 and GM-CSF for GM-CFU Synergizes with CSF-1 for HPP-CFC
rhGM-CSF	GM-CFU G-CFU Mega-CFU BFU-E (with Epo) Blast colony Small cell lung line HL-60 AML progenitors Eosinophils	Some myeloid leukemia cell lines	Enhances cytotoxic activity Enhances phagocytosis Enhances ADCC Increases cell adhesion protein expression (Mo-1) Enhances superoxide and hydrogen peroxide production Inhibits neutrophil motility (NIF-T) Increases arachidonic acid release Increases leukotriene B$_4$ synthesis Increases synthesis of membrane protein Increases synthesis of nucleoprotein Enhances eosinophil cytotoxicity Promotes murine placental growth	Induces intracellular accumulation of TNF and IL-1 Modulates transdown of receptors
rhM-CSF	M-CFU GM-CFU G-CFU	Monocytes	Supports survival of differentiated macrophages *in vitro* Decreases protein catabolism (at low doses) Increases protein synthesis and proliferation (at high doses) Increases macrophage antitumor activity Increases oxygen radical secretion Increases plasminogen activator secretion Interacts with c-fms product	Synergizes with low levels of GM-CSF to increase M-CFU Interacts less clearly with GM-CSF, G-CSF, and IL-3
rhIL-3	G-CFU GM-CFU M-CFU Eosinophils Mast cells Natural-killer-like cells BFU-E Mixed CFU AML blast progenitors HPP-CFC (with M-CSF)	?	Alters calcium mobilization Induces 2-hydroxy steroid dehydrogenase Induces Thy-1 expression Translocates protein kinase C (?)	
rhIL-1	With M-CSF and IL-3 = hemopoietin-1	T-cells Fibroblast/glial cells Mesangial cells Synovial cells	Induces neutrophia Activates chondrocytes Enhances chemotaxis for monocytes and neutrophils	Induces GM-CSF production Induces IL-2 production Increases prostaglandin synthesis Augments B-cell response

[1]CSF, colony-stimulating factor. [2]rhG-CSF, recombinant human granulocyte CSF; rhGM-CSF, recombinant human granulocyte-macrophage CSF; rhM-CSF, recombinant human macrophage CSF; rhIL-3, recombinant human interleukin-3; rhIL-1, recombinant human interleukin-1. [3]CFU, colony-forming unit; G-CFU, granulocyte CFU; GM-CFU, granulocyte-macrophage CFU; M-CFU, macrophage CFU; Mega-CFU, megakaryocyte CFU; BFU-E (with Epo), burst-forming unit-erythroid (with erythropoietin); AML, acute myelogenous leukemia; M-CFU, macrophage CFU; HPP-CFC, high proliferative potential colony-forming cells; M-CSF, macrophage colony-stimulating factor; IL-3, interleukin-3. [4]ADCC, antibody-dependent cellular cytotoxicity; NIF-T, neutrophil migration inhibition factor. [5]TNF, tumor necrosis factor.

radiation-injured patients. For example, Weisbart and his colleagues have demonstrated that rhGM-CSF is equivalent to neutrophil migration inhibition factor (NIF-T) and is responsible for inhibiting neutrophil migration *in vitro*. This effect is presumably important in keeping cells at a local site of inflammation so that phagocytosis can be enhanced. In addition, GM-CSF has been shown to have significant chemotactic properties, attracting neutrophils to an area in a concentration-dependent manner. An inflammatory response to an infection requires that neutrophils be attracted and then anchored to a given site; then, phagocytosis and intracellular killing of ingested organisms must occur. If GM-CSF circulates at all, only low levels are present; detailed studies of the pharmacology of GM-CSF have not been performed, however.

On the other hand, G-CSF has not been reported to have neutrophil migration-inhibiting properties. We and others have reported that similar effects occur *in vivo* during systemic treatment with rhGM-CSF and rhG-CSF in the transplant setting.

Biochemical evaluations *in vitro* suggest that different doses may be effective for enhancing proliferative effects and for enhancing functional capacity of neutrophils. Enhanced neutrophil function occurs at very low doses of the recombinant growth factors, but the effects on enhanced proliferation appear to require significantly higher dosages. It is not yet clear whether there is a bell-shaped curve to the effects on functional capacity or whether enhanced doses of the recombinant growth factors may, in fact, limit or inhibit the effects on enhancement of neutrophil function. Bell-shaped dose-response curves have been reported for other human proteins, such as alpha interferon; such effects would not be unexpected.

Cytokine Cascades

The hematopoietic CSF's appear to be interrelated in an extremely intricate manner. CSF's have been able to enhance their own production, for example, in the case of IL-1 (autocrine), as well as to induce the enhanced intracellular accumulation and release of other cytokines. GM-CSF has been shown to enhance production of both G-CSF and M-CSF, and IL-1 enhances production of G-CSF, GM-CSF, and M-CSF as well.

The relationship between the CSF's may, in fact, be even more complex. GM-CSF has been demonstrated to increase the intracellular accumulation of tumor necrosis factor (TNF). Although the release of TNF from cells that have been stimulated by GM-CSF does not appear to occur spontaneously, the addition of a second factor, such as endotoxin or lipopolysaccharide, will result in the release of significant quantities of TNF from stimulated cells. These cytokine cascades may be complicated, and the interactions between the CSF's are complicated and incompletely understood.

Clinical Effects of Colony-Stimulating Factors

Several CSF's have entered clinical trials, and the evolution of clinical effects with other CSF's is just beginning. RhG-CSF and rhGM-CSF have both been studied in bone marrow transplant settings, in patients receiving chemotherapy, and in patients being treated for myelodysplasia, aplastic anemia, and other bone marrow failure states. These clinical observations have a direct bearing on the use of recombinant growth factors in the treatment of patients with radiation injuries, particularly in bone marrow transplantation, in which hematopoietic recovery occurs from the infused stem cells, and in chemotherapy-induced injury, in which dose-related inhibitions of myelopoiesis are seen. Extrapolation to potential effects in the radiation injury setting might be considered. Although associated with significant clinical side effects at high doses, the CSF's can be used effectively at much lower doses with clinically acceptable toxicity.

The clinical experience with the CSF's, however, is notable for several features. First, it is clear from evaluations of the effects of the CSF's on bone marrow that improved marrow cellularity enhances myelopoiesis. However, a variety of clinical and *in vitro* data suggest that the CSF's currently in clinical testing require the presence of a committed progenitor on which they can work. GM-CSF and G-CSF generally do not seem to affect the pluripotent stem cell but rather exert their effects on a committed progenitor, enhancing its proliferation and differentiation into a mature neutrophil. These effects have important implications for use in radiation injury, because radiation doses capable of destroying marrow stem cells are unlikely to be helped by the intensive use of CSF's if there are few stem cells remaining. The only solution in this setting is to provide the radiation victim with acceptable marrow, or at least with marrow progenitors, on which the CSF's can act. If the radiation exposure has been sufficiently low that marrow has not been ablated, use of the CSF's may be valuable.

One factor that has not been discussed thus far is the impact of the injury on the bone marrow microenvironment. The use of the CSF's implies that there is a specific, or at least a pharmacologic, deficit of a particular CSF. In the setting of severe injury, radiation or otherwise, production of the other endogenous cytokines likely has been affected as well. Hence, the systematic administration of a single CSF may be ineffective in producing the optimal, or even the desired, effect. Clinical usage of multiple CSF's is only beginning, however, and the final utility of these investigations to the treatment of radiation injury is unclear. However, the use of CSF's with radiation-injured patients is a rapidly evolving field, and individuals with significant experience in the use of the CSF's should be called in early.

It does not appear at present that the CSF's in clinical usage (G-CSF and GM-CSF) are capable of exhausting the marrow progenitor cells. Clinical and experimental data argue that these factors are sufficiently restricted to mature progenitors and that they will not deplete the body of the appropriate marrow stem cells. However, the use will clearly accelerate the proliferation and release of compounds into the periphery.

Two features are notable in our studies of hematopoietic reconstitution following high-dose cyclophosphamide, cisplatin and carmustine (BCNU), and autologous bone marrow support in patients being treated for breast cancer or melanoma. Compared to control patients, who historically did not receive CSF, the interval before the first appearance of neutrophilic granulocytes is the same, but once cells begin to appear, the slope of recovery and the number of cells appearing in circulation are enhanced. This effect does not appear to be the result of redistribution of the neutrophils but rather represents enhanced production and release of mature cells from the bone marrow. However, there is also substantial heterogeneity in the responses of individual patients to both rhGM-CSF and rhG-CSF. Patients who previously received extensive chemotherapy had less proliferative effect from a given dose of recombinant growth factor than previously untreated patients. Patients in whom marrow purging with 4-hydroperoxycyclophosphamide has been undertaken and who have been treated with rhGM-CSF during recovery have only a limited effect from the treatment with rhGM-CSF. Again, this finding suggests that the CSF's require adequate marrow progenitors to work optimally.

Recent data on the administration of rhGM-CSF to patients with graft failure have suggested a more complex response in marrow-deficient states. In this setting, patients who have received rhGM-CSF after autologous or allogeneic bone marrow transplantation fails to produce an adequate marrow graft appear, at least in some cases, to respond with sustained myelopoiesis to a short-term course of recombinant myeloid growth factor. This sustained recovery occurs despite only a short-term use of the recombinant growth factor. The mechanism for this effect is not understood, but presumably involves the stimulation of some autocrine function associated with enhanced marrow proliferation. Whether this effect is seen with CSF's other than GM-CSF is unknown. The requirement of GM-CSF and G-CSF for mature progenitors on which to work suggests an alternative mechanism by which the use of CSF's may be facilitated in the setting of a radiation injury. Granulocyte transfusions have, in general, not been widely used because the short half-life of the granulocytes limits their value. However, recent experiences at several laboratories suggest that both rhGM-CSF and rhG-CSF can enhance the number of mature progenitors in the peripheral blood. Techniques for harvesting these peripheral blood progenitor cells using continuous-flow pheresis have been detailed, and may serve as a source of progenitors with which mature growth factors could be used as an adjunct in radiation accident patients. The administration of these cell products, coupled with the administration of the recombinant growth factor, may allow these committed progenitors to proliferate into an enhanced number of neutrophilic granulocytes, enabling more effective treatment of infectious disorders. This approach is as yet untested and may be associated with significant toxicity (as allogeneic granulocyte transfusions were in the past).

Use of Growth Factor in Radiation Injury

The clinical use of the CSF's is in its infancy, and only the most general recommendations can be made based on current data. Further, the understanding of biological and clinical effects of the CSF's is changing rapidly. Clearly, any recommendation regarding the use of CSF's in the radiation accident victim depends on accurate dosimetry. The primary consideration is to remove the patient from continued radiation exposure; if the radiation exposure is ongoing, the CSF's likely should not be employed, based on current assessment. Although there is little evidence that the CSF's will induce the stem cell to produce mature progenitors, theoretical concerns suggest that one might be able to induce stem cells into cycle, or at least into an enhanced proliferative state, which would increase potentially their sensitivity to radiation injury. Indeed, other factors, such as gamma interferon, may be used in shutting down marrow activity at this point, in an attempt to minimize ongoing radiation injury. Hence, accurate dosimetry and removal of the patient from any source of radiation should follow radiation injury as soon as possible. Tissue deposition of isotopes, such as cesium-137, that might provide ongoing radiation exposure should be measured carefully.

Experimental data from animal models suggest that the use of IL-1 immediately following radiation exposure may protect animals from lethal myelosuppression. Early studies suggest that this approach may be true in primates as well. Studies in humans have not been undertaken. Canine experience suggests that in sublethally irradiated animals the use of G-CSF may protect animals from infection or other causes of death by enhancing proliferation and maturation of myeloid precursors. In the first few days after acute radiation injury, all data seem to point to the early use of the CSF's; G-CSF and GM-CSF appear to be the most likely candidates for early use. However, consideration of other factors, such as the extent of burns or other infectious complications, may mitigate the choice of particular agents. The decrease in neutrophil migration to sites of soft-tissue infection suggests that GM-CSF in the setting of severe burns might be less effective than G-CSF. However, in patients with extensive gastrointestinal injury, whose primary problem is sepsis, the presence of large numbers of activated neutrophils in the systemic circulation may be valuable, thus the use of GM-CSF may be appropriate. In the radiation injury setting, each patient must be monitored individually for the effects and toxicities of the recombinant growth factors.

Based on experience in the graft-failure following allogeneic and autologous bone marrow transplantation, patients who remain severely myelosuppressed several weeks after exposure to radiation might be considered for a treatment of rhGM-CSF. Although this treatment setting has not been fully explored, the ability of rhGM-CSF to enhance sustained myelopoiesis in patients with graft failure after bone marrow transplantation argues for its use in this generally life-threatening situation.

Because clinical experience with the CSF's is limited, full recommendations for their use in particular settings cannot be made at this time. Clearly, the induction of other cytokines may play a major role in the radiation injury victim. The systemic stress of the injury or associated infections may induce TNF, IL-1, or other cytokines. Depending on the extent of the injury to the cells responsible for production of these cytokines, they may interact with the pharmacologic administration of any of the CSF's used to enhance hematopoiesis. Such interactions may be either positive or negative and should be considered carefully.

Finally, the effect of the radiation injury on the marrow stroma is of major clinical importance. It appears that the normal development of marrow requires an appropriately functioning microenvironment in which the hematopoietic stem cells are provided and the stromal cells are functional. Current biological evidence suggests that the marrow stroma is relatively radiation resistant and that local or immediate injury is less likely to the stromal cells than to the proliferating marrow progenitors. The effects on marrow stroma more likely will be seen later.

Dysfunction in the coordinated secretion of the appropriate cytokines may well be expected, and as the understanding of the clinical use of the various cytokines improves, manipulation of the administration of several of the CSF's may be appropriately considered. Selection of the cytokine to be used in a particular clinical setting depends on an understanding of the functional enhancement that one wants to achieve. Clearly, these areas require substantial continued investigation.

Conclusion

Recent molecular cloning, *in vitro* expression, and formulation of the recombinant CSF's offer a potential tool for aiding victims of radiation injury. Enhancing the rate of marrow proliferation in patients with sublethally injured marrow may improve the time of hematopoietic recovery sufficiently to save some patients from death due to the hematopoietic injury and its associated infectious and organ system complications. The field is yet in its infancy, and full understanding of the use of CSF's requires further clinical investigation. Nonetheless, response teams for radiation injury accidents should include individuals with expertise in the use of CSF's.

Consensus Summary Statement on the Treatment of Radiation Injuries

Introduction

The radiation environment during a nuclear accident or disaster is likely to be uncontrolled and ill defined. This was emphasized by the three most recent accidents—the reactor explosion in Chernobyl, U.S.S.R. (1986); the internal and external exposure of victims to cesium-137 in Goiânia, Brazil (1987); and the exposure of workers in a radiation sterilization facility in San Salvador, El Salvador (1989). The radiation may differ in quality, energy, and dose rate. The exposure may be nonuniform and heterogeneous, and may involve only part of the body, depending on the location, position, and movement of the subjects relative to the radiation source and available shielding. Physicians treating irradiated patients may find that patients have also been traumatized by burns and/or wounds.

Many individuals who have received total-body radiation doses that lie within the range that causes the hematopoietic syndrome will require intensive medical care. The patient with combined injuries—one who has been traumatized as well as irradiated—will require additional care for the associated trauma and consequent immunosuppression. The ill-defined and uncontrolled nature of radiation exposure and nuclear accidents usually forecasts a nonuniform exposure, with the variable dose distribution suggesting a possible sparing of some bone marrow and/or gastrointestinal stem cells. With this in mind, it is possible that recovery may occur even when radiation doses extend well into the lethal range of the hematopoietic and gastrointestinal syndromes.

Success with therapeutic regimens of replacement (platelets, fluids, and electrolytes) and substitution (antibiotics) supports the concept that infection and hemorrhage are the primary factors in the lethal consequences of radiation exposure in the hematopoietic syndrome. The practical application of these concepts depends on the fact that damage to the stem cell system is reversible; the surviving fraction of hematopoietic stem cells must be capable of spontaneous regeneration. These supportive and maintenance therapies were successfully used after the nuclear disaster in Chernobyl. Patients with clinical manifestations of the acute radiation syndrome were treated using isolation, antimicrobial decontamination of the intestine, systemic antibiotics, and transfusions of red blood cells and platelets. Supportive procedures for empirical anti-infection treatment were highly effective. There were practically no deaths caused solely by infection among patients experiencing acute radiation sickness.

The immediate treatment of associated injuries is a primary determinant of survival. The degree of radiation-induced marrow aplasia (reversible or irreversible) may not be known for days because of the uncontrolled nature of the exposure and its potential to be nonuniform and heterogeneous. These facts make reliance on a physical dose estimate impossible and underscore the need for monitoring biological parameters to estimate the severity of injuries and the probability of survival. Reliable triage and good clinical care based on comprehensive biological data will ensure the best chance for casualty recovery should a critical number of stem cells survive the radiation exposure.

Data for uncomplicated human radiation exposures within the hematopoietic syndrome range are relatively limited. The evidence (exclusive of the three recent accidents) comes from five primary sources: (1) persons exposed to the nuclear weapons detonations in Hiroshima and Nagasaki, (2) radiotherapy of persons with Ewing's sarcoma with therapeutic total-body bilateral exposure to gamma radiation, (3) two nuclear accidents (Vinca, Yugoslavia, and Oak Ridge, TN) involving nine people exposed to mixed neutron and gamma radiations, (4) two radiation accidents (New Jersey) involving two people exposed to cobalt-60 radiation, and (5) bone marrow transplant recipients receiving total-body radiation. Information collected from these exposures, the three recent radiation accidents, and experimental data provide a basis for a consensus on the treatment of radiation injuries.

Consensus on a Treatment Protocol

Three panels were established to develop a consensus on treatment of hematopoietic injury, infectious complications, and combined injury, the topics discussed at the First Consensus Development Conference on the Treatment of Radiation Injuries, Washington, DC, May 10-13, 1989. Each panel presented a summary of its discussion on a specified treatment area. Figure 1 provides a protocol for the treatment of radiation injuries, summarized from the deliberations of the three panels. The outlined protocol for the treatment of radiation injuries is based on uniform total-body radiation exposure, and may not be applicable in all accident or mass casualty situations.

Based on the severity of the radiation exposure, casualties can be classified into four treatment categories: mild, moderate, severe, and lethal. A consensus was not reached on the specific dose ranges for these categories, primarily because of the difficulty in converting an air dose to a meaningful tissue dose. Nevertheless, dose ranges are indicated in figure 1. The main goal of this classification system is to increase the likelihood of survival. In treating the casualty, not the radiation dose, the most reliable guide is the change in levels of blood cells and cytogenetics.

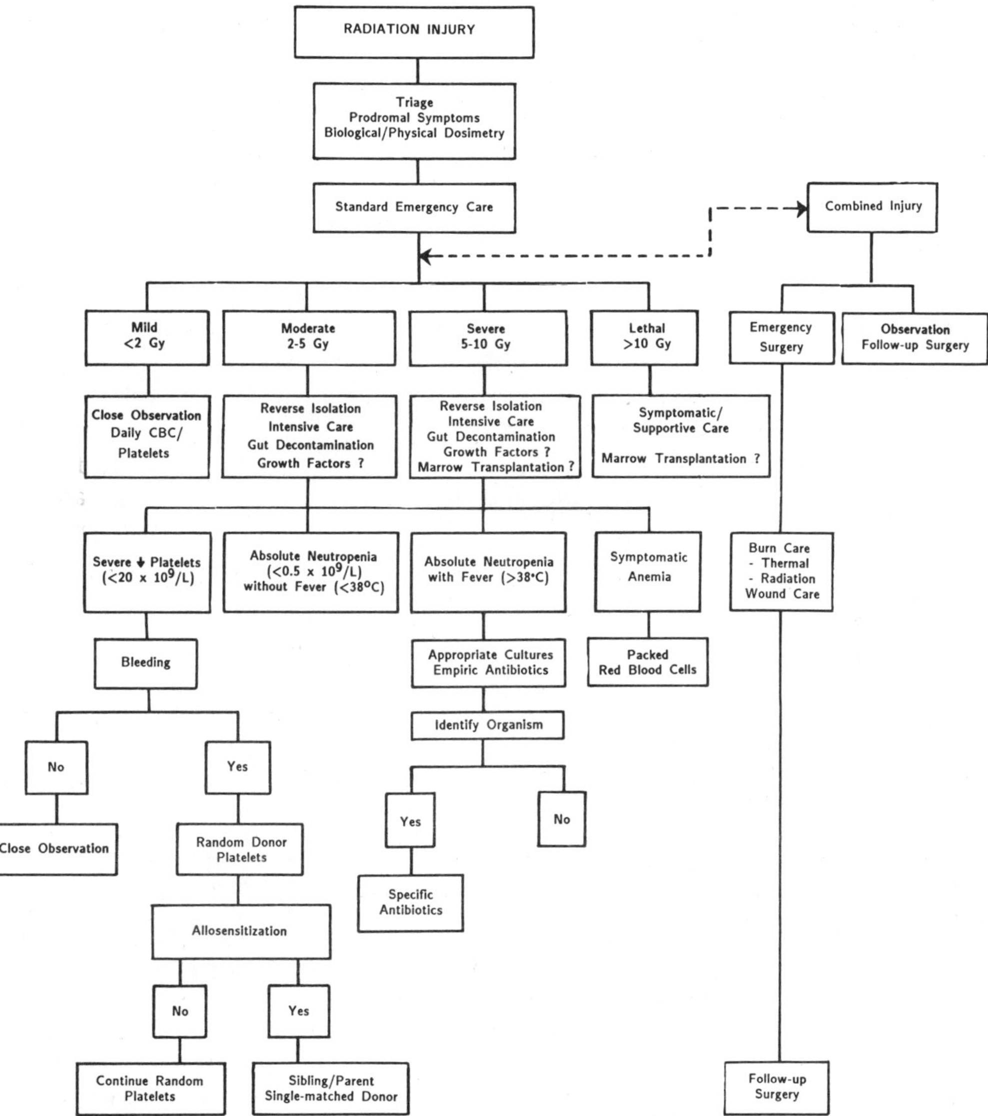

Figure 1. Treatment schema. The outlined protocol for treatment of radiation injuries is based on uniform total-body radiation exposure, and may not be applicable in all accident or mass casualty situations.

Medical Management of Radiation Injuries

The following combines common areas and emphasizes specific requirements for three stages of managing injuries. The medical management of radiation and/or combined injuries can be divided into three stages: triage, emergency care, and definitive care (table 1). Quality care can be given when there are few casualties, and care can be provided in a well-equipped facility. The therapeutic modalities to be implemented vary according to current medical knowledge and experience. Precisely implemented modalities will depend on

Table 1. Personnel and Data Required for the Medical Management of a Radiation Accident

Stages of medical management	Personnel[1]	Data
Triage	Triage director Radiation safety officer Support personnel	Dosimetry (when available) History[2]

Emergency care
Resuscitation
	Physician
	Nurse
	Radiation safety officer
	Support personnel
		Biological samples
		Exposure estimation
		Contamination evaluation
		Patient care
		Infectious disease
		  surveillance
		Acute radiation syndrome
		  flowchart

Surgery	Surgeon and assistants Anesthesiologist Nurses Radiation safety officer	Patient monitoring Acute radiation syndrome flowchart

Definitive care	Surgery team
	Hematologist
	Infectious disease
	 specialist
	Consultants
	  Endocrinologist
	  Dermatologist
	  Radiobiologist
	  Psychologist
	  Nutritionist
		Biological samples
		Patient care
		Hematologic monitoring
		Infectious disease
		  surveillance
		Acute radiation syndrome
		  flowchart

[1]Personnel involved in triage and emergency care must be monitored for radiation exposure and rotated frequently, whenever possible.
[2]Presence of symptoms such as emesis, erythema, and diarrhea must be emphasized.

the number of casualties, available medical facilities, and resources. The panel concurred that the recommendations for treatment of a few casualties may not be applicable for treatment of mass casualties because of limited resources.

Triage

During the triage stage, the triage director can categorize victims by degree of injury from trauma, radiation, or their combination, and can estimate chances for survival. Triage is extremely important in mass casualty situations that require allocation of limited medical resources to those who require treatment and have the best chances of survival. There is no immediate life-threatening hazard from a dose of radiation alone that is survivable. Treat the associated injuries first.

An acute radiation syndrome flowchart for each patient should be maintained. This flowchart provides continuity throughout prolonged therapy that may be delivered by various caretakers and in different facilities.

Estimating the degree of radiation damage and exposure is difficult. Prodromal symptoms, which begin within hours of exposure, are characterized by gastrointestinal and neurovascular signs and symptoms, including nausea, vomiting, diarrhea, fatigue, weakness, fever, and headache. The gastrointestinal symptoms generally do not last longer than 24-48 hours after exposure. The time of onset, severity, and duration of these signs are dose dependent and dose-rate dependent, and should be used in conjunction with early biological parameters, such as granulocyte and lymphocyte levels, to determine the presence and severity of the acute radiation syndrome. These signs and symptoms must be used initially to determine if the casualty is one that is related to radiation exposure.

The rate and degree of decrease in blood cells are dose dependent. Blood samples should be taken daily during the first 2 weeks. A useful rule of thumb is: if lymphocytes have decreased by 50 percent and are less than $1 \times 10^9/$ L within 24-48 hours, the patient has received at least a moderate dose of radiation. In combined injuries, lymphocytes may be an unreliable indicator. Patients with severe burns and/or trauma to more than one system often develop lymphopenia. Associated injuries (trauma/burn) should be assessed by standard procedures, keeping in mind that the signs and symptoms of tissue injuries can mimic and obscure those caused by acute radiation effects.

Effective triage relies on accurate analysis of early signs and symptoms, substantiated by biological parameters associated with radiation exposure. Treatment must be determined after assessing the radiation injury and the indicated therapies for the type of organ damage. Conventional injuries that are benign by themselves can become lethal when combined with radiation exposure.

Emergency Care

Following a radiation accident, injured persons should be stabilized (intravenous fluids, bandages, and ventilatory support provided) at the site before transport to treatment centers within the local area for further evaluation and treatment. Those with trauma and burns and without radiation injury (determined by their location at the time of the accident or by the lack of general prodromal symptoms, such as nausea and vomiting) should be referred to specialized treatment centers according to their injuries. Patients who probably suffered from radiation injury (identified by signs and symptoms) should be referred to treatment centers that can evaluate and treat bone marrow failure. Radiation injuries, burns, or multiple trauma will be treated at these centers by a team (table 1). Treatment should be managed by representatives from hematology, infectious disease, surgery, and psychiatry services. Other centers should be alerted to the possible need for platelets and red cells, and should verify that all blood products have been irradiated. Hospitals in the vicinity should be alerted about the possible need for supplies and blood products.

Definitive Care of Hematopoietic Injury

Platelet support. The requirement for platelet support depends on the patient's condition. In irradiated patients with or without other major medical problems (infection, gastrointestinal problems, or trauma), the platelets should be maintained at greater than 20×10^9/L. If surgery is needed, the platelet count should be greater than 75×10^9/L.

Limited platelet support is likely to come from random donors. Should refractoriness develop, family members as well as HLA-compatible donors from the general population can be considered as platelet donors. The use of platelet products from which white blood cells have been removed is desirable to minimize both allosensitization and the risk of transmission of viral illnesses, such as cytomegalovirus. All blood products should receive 15-20 Gy of radiation before infusion to prevent graft-versus-host disease through infusion of mononuclear cells present in the products. If a transplant is to be performed, the use of platelets from related donors should be avoided.

Growth factors. Hematopoietic growth factors, such as granulocyte colony-stimulating factor (G-CSF) and granulocyte-macrophage colony-stimulating factor (GM-CSF), are potent stimulators of hematopoiesis. Preclinical studies in nonhuman primates, mice, and dogs demonstrate an increase in radiation survival with G-CSF and GM-CSF treatment. A similar effect may occur in humans. Definitive trials of growth factors in victims of radiation accidents are not possible, but ongoing phase II and phase III clinical trials in patients with bone marrow failure or after autologous or allogeneic marrow grafting will further define the risks and benefits of these factors. Studies of other potentially useful growth factors, such as interleukin-1 and interleukin-3, may delineate the potential use of these cytokines as well.

Consideration must be given to the type of radiation exposure (internal or external), the presence of nonhematopoietic organ injury, and the radioisotope. Growth factor therapy may not be helpful, and may be detrimental where there is prolonged internal irradiation by long-lived isotopes. Potential risks include acceleration of leukemogenesis and prevention of neutrophil migration into soft tissues. Early granulocyte recovery following growth factor therapy may indicate lower-than-estimated radiation dose exposure.

Based on current data, use of G-CSF or GM-CSF is reasonable for victims of radiation injury who have received a dose sufficient to cause prolonged neutropenia but not to prevent eventual bone marrow recovery. This dose is unknown, but a reasonable approximation might be 4-8 Gy of uniform total-body exposure.

Data on growth factors administered to accidentally irradiated humans is limited (13 cases in 3 accidents), and in each case, administration occurred at 1 week or more postirradiation. In 11 cases, the growth factor was administered about 3-5 weeks postexposure. In the 13 cases, results have not yielded data that could be evaluated. Earlier administration of growth factors (1-3 days postexposure) may prove more beneficial in inducing granulocytosis.

Bone marrow transplantation. Total-body irradiation produces dose-dependent toxicity to the bone marrow. Increasing doses lead to more protracted pancytopenia and increasing risk of death from infection and/or hemorrhage. The dose of radiation to the bone marrow that would effectively prevent recovery within a period required for survival is unknown.

A reasonable estimate for an LD_{50} in humans receiving clinical support is 6 Gy free in air. The use of broad spectrum antibiotics, blood product support, and perhaps hematopoietic growth factors may give a possible chance of surviving an 8-Gy dose of radiation. Experimental animal data suggest that marrow transplantation from an HLA-identical sibling should be considered, even at doses of uniform total-body radiation as low as 5 Gy. To prevent transplant-related complications, such as graft-versus-host disease, one may consider depleting the bone marrow of T-lymphocytes. However, the transplanted bone marrow may only engraft transiently until autologous marrow function recovers. Exposure doses of 5-6 Gy will likely prevent permanent engraftment.

The timing of marrow grafting is crucial and presents a dilemma. Animal data suggest that the marrow should be infused within the first 3-5 days of radiation exposure. This coincides with the peak period of immunosuppression, and graft rejection, therefore, will be less likely. These findings stress the importance of developing reliable clinical and laboratory parameters to assess the degree of radiation damage to the marrow as quickly as possible and to determine which patients should be given marrow transplants. Waiting for a week or longer after the radiation exposure would require some form of immunosuppressive treatment to prepare the patient for a marrow graft. Such treatment may be less tolerated by the patient who is a radiation accident victim. The marrow transplant must be carried out at a treatment facility equipped for such procedures.

Definitive Care of Infectious Complications

This report addresses infectious complications that occur in profoundly neutropenic patients ($< 0.1 \times 10^9$/L neutrophils). Those with lesser degrees of neutropenia are at substantially less risk of infection and hence do not require the vigorous prevention and treatment modality described here. These patients may also have traumatic injuries that can aggravate their prognoses. Treatment of these combined injuries may require more aggressive interventions. It must be kept in mind that management of traumatic injuries and restoration of bone marrow cellularity are essential to survival. Interventions to reduce and control infections will help ensure survival during the immunocompromised state associated with this repair process.

Therapeutic options were classified as prevention and management of infections. The recommendations may be modified to simplify their application in situations that involve many patients.

Prevention of infection. Table 2 shows approaches to prevent infection. Initial care of medical casualties with moderate and severe radiation exposure should probably include early institution of measures to reduce pathogen acquisition, with emphasis on low-microbial-content food, acceptable water supplies, frequent hand washing (or wearing gloves), and air filtration. Prophylactic use of selective gut decontamination with antibiotics that suppress aerobes but preserve anaerobes is recommended. These measures help control the alimentary canal source (mouth, esophagus, and intestines) of postinjury infections. Maintenance of gastric acidity (avoidance of antacids and H_2 blockers) may prevent bacteria from colonizing and invading the gastric mucosa and may reduce the frequency of nosocomial pneumonia due to aspiration

Table 2. Proposed Approaches to Prevent Infection in Immunocompromised Patients

Reduction of invasive procedures (for example, nasogastric tubes) and development of colonization-resistant inert surfaces

Reduction of microbial acquisition

    Contact control (for example, handwashing)
    Water treatment (when indicated)
    Food (low microbial diet)
    Air control to reduce *Aspergillus* infections (useful if available)

Suppression of microorganisms

    Total microbial suppression (not recommended because of suppression of anaerobes)

    Selective decontamination
      Administer oral nonabsorbable antibacterials (for example, quinolones) that preserve anaerobic bacteria; nystatin
      Anthelmintics if indicated
      Observe for resistant bacterial acquisition during clinical course

    Antivirals (acyclovir) as guided by positive anti-HSV (herpes simplex virus) antibody or empirically if test not available

    Physiological interventions
    Maintain gastric acidity
      Avoid antacids and H_2 blockers
      Use sucralfate for stress ulcer prophylaxis when indicated to reduce gastric colonization and pneumonia
    Provide early oral enteral nutrition, when feasible

    Adequate personal hygiene
    Povidone-iodine (Betadine™) or chlorhexidine for skin disinfection
    Shampoo
    Oral hygiene (brushing and flossing)

Improvement of host defenses

    Active vaccination for expected pathogens (for example, influenza)
    Passive immunization with immunoglobulins (utility not established to date)
    Immunomodulators (for example, glucan and trehalose dimycolate)
      (utility not established in humans)
      Can enhance macrophage antibacterial activity prior to marrow recovery
      May enhance effectiveness of subsequently administered growth factors
      Could be simple to use (one administration orally)

---

of these organisms. The use of sucralfate or prostaglandin analogues may prevent gastric hemorrhage without decreasing gastric activity. When possible, early oral feeding is preferred to intravenous feeding to maintain the immunologic and physiologic integrity of the gut. Surgical implantation of a subcutaneously tunneled central venous catheter should be considered to allow frequent venous access. Meticulous attention to proper care is necessary to reduce catheter-associated infections.

Management of infection. The management of established or suspected infection (neutropenia and fever) in irradiated persons is similar to that used in other febrile neutropenic patients. First, an empirical regimen of antibiotics should be selected, based on the pattern of bacterial susceptibility and nosocomial infections in the particular institution and the degree of neutropenia. Combination antibiotic therapy (extended spectrum beta-lactam (penicillin or cephalosporin) plus aminoglycoside ± vancomycin) for initial therapy of patients with profound neutropenia (< 0.1 x 10^9/L neutrophils) is recommended. Monotherapy (ceftazidime or imipenem) is appropriate for patients with less intense neutropenia.

Modifications of this initial antibiotic regimen should include a thorough evaluation of the history, physical findings, laboratory data (including chest radiograph), and epidemiological information. Antifungal coverage with amphotericin B should be added, if indicated, for patients who remain persistently febrile for 7 days or more on antibiotic therapy in association with clinical evidence of infection, or if they have new fever on or after day 7 of treatment with antibiotics. If there is evidence of resistant gram-positive infection, vancomycin should be added.

Surveillance cultures may be useful for monitoring acquisition of resistant bacteria during prophylaxis and emergence of fungi. A once or twice weekly sampling of surveillance cultures from natural orifices and skin folds (for example, axillae, groin) would be reasonable, but should be modified based on the institutional patterns of nosocomial infections.

Definitive Care of Combined Injury

Combined injury is defined as a concurrent trauma (mechanical or thermal) and radiation injury occurring during a period of time before recovery from any one of the injuries. Combined injury may afflict variable numbers of casualties. Because radiation injury is not immediately life threatening, initial care should address the associated conventional injuries, for example, thermal burns and wounds. The emergency medical procedures for ventilation, perfusion, and hemorrhage should be provided first, and then casualties should be stabilized. After stabilization, radioisotope decontamination should be performed before emergency surgery, definitive care, and treatment of radiation injuries. Collection of biological samples during the resuscitation stages will supplement the initial data collected during triage.

Ideally, definitive care should immediately follow resuscitation. However, in mass casualty situations with limited resources, the assessment made during triage would indicate which individuals would benefit the most from immediate surgery, and those who would benefit from observation and standard medical therapy. During the definitive care stage, the assistance of various medical specialists and consultants is desired, especially in managing difficult cases (table 1). In mass casualty situations, however, the primary caretaker (any trained or untrained individual) should be capable of providing basic therapies.

There may be many psychological problems accompanying radiation accidents. Professional help may be necessary to treat these problems.

Surgical procedures play a part in both emergency care and definitive care of patients with combined injuries. Recognizing the difficulties associated with the management of soft tissue wounds, serious consideration should be given to alternative ways to close the wound, for example, biological wound coverings and skin grafts. Surgical correction of life-threatening and other major injuries should be carried out as soon as possible (within 36-48 hours); elective procedures should be postponed until late in the convalescent period (45-60 days) following hematopoietic recovery.

Treatment of thermal burns should include early excision of potentially septic tissue and closure of the wounds, preferably by skin grafting. Radiation burns and thermal burns should be treated differently, especially when using surgery, which should be delayed in the case of radiation burns. Information on the specific treatment of radiation burns to the skin is currently not available.

The closure of the traumatic wound, which generally should be attempted as soon as possible, emerges as the most challenging of all surgical therapeutic efforts in the treatment of the patient with combined injuries because of the relatively short period following injury when surgery can be performed safely. This narrow time frame results from the radiation-induced suppression of cellular elements necessary for wound healing. The following procedures are recommended after resuscitation and emergency surgery: (1) return the patient to the operating room within 48 hours, obtain quantitative bacterial cultures, and, if the wound is clinically clean, graft all defects with autologous skin; (2) remove dressings at 96-120 hours, and, if the wounds have been appropriately debrided, skin grafts should have closed the wounds; and (3) if additional debridement is necessary at 48 hours, the previous procedures should begin again at 96 hours.

Appendixes

Appendix A

Consensus Panel Participants

Hematopoietic Injury Complications: Eugene P. Cronkite, M.D. (moderator); Rainer Storb, M.D.; Richard Champlin, M.D.; C. Robert Valeri, M.D.; Joseph Laver, M.D.; Thomas J. MacVittie, Ph.D.; Joseph H. Antin, M.D.; Robert Peter Gale, M.D.; and Dorothee Krumwieh, M.D.

Infectious Complications: Richard I. Walker, Ph.D., and Itzhak Brook, M.D. (moderators); Stephen C. Schimpff, M.D.; Alexandre R. Oliveira, M.D.; Gary P. Zaloga, M.D.; Thomas J. Walsh, M.D.; and Anna Butturini, M.D.

Combined Injury Complications: Robert W. Young, Ph.D. (moderator); Erwin F. Hirsch, M.D.; William K. Becker, M.D.; Patricia M. Mertz; G. David Ledney, Ph.D.; and Robert C. Ricks, Ph.D.

Appendix B

Conference Participants

Joseph Harry Antin, M.D.
Division of Hematology
Department of Medicine
Brigham and Women's Hospital
Boston, MA 02115

Yoshiro Aoki, M.D.
National Institute of Radiological Sciences
4-9-1, Anagawa
Chiba City, Japan 260

Sharon Aukerman, Ph.D.
Cetus Corporation
1400 53rd Street
Emeryville, CA 94608

Michael K. Bamat, Ph.D.
Pro-Neuron, Inc.
1500 E. Jefferson Street
Rockville, MD 20852

Siegmund J. Baum, Ph.D.
6600 Greyswood Road
Bethesda, MD 20817

William K. Becker, M.D.
LTC, MC, USA
U.S. Army Institute of Surgical Research
Fort Sam Houston, TX 78234-5012

Mary Ellen Berger, Ed.D., RN
Radiation Emergency Assistance
   Center/Training Site
P.O. Box 117
Oak Ridge, TN 37831-0117

William F. Blakely, Ph.D.
Radiation Biochemistry Department
Armed Forces Radiobiology Research Institute
Bethesda, MD 20814-5145

Itzhak Brook, M.D.
CDR, MC, USN
Experimental Hematology Department
Armed Forces Radiobiology Research Institute
Bethesda, MD 20814-5145

Byron Brown, M.D.
3361 Fandanso Place
Las Vegas, NV 89102

Doris Browne, M.D., MPH
LTC, MC, USA
Military Requirements and
   Applications Department
Armed Forces Radiobiology Research Institute
Bethesda, MD 20814-5145

Bruce M. Burnett, Ph.D.
U.S. Food and Drug Administration (HFZ-60)
5600 Fishers Lane
Rockville, MD 20857

Jerrold Bushberg, Ph.D.
Assistant Professor of Radiology
Technical Director of Nuclear Medicine
University of California
Davis Medical Center
2315 Stockton Boulevard
Sacramento, CA 95817

Anna Butturini, M.D.
Department of Pediatrics
University of Parma
Parma, 43100 Italy

George Catravas, Ph.D.
Chair of Science
Armed Forces Radiobiology Research Institute
Bethesda, MD 20814-5145

Richard E. Champlin, M.D.
Division of Hematology/Oncology
Department of Medicine
Jonsson Comprehensive Cancer Center
School of Medicine
University of California
Los Angeles, CA 90024

Raymond L. Chaput, Ph.D.
CAPT, MSC, USN
Naval Medical Command (MEDCOM-26)
Washington, DC 20372-5201

Sarah H. Comley, Ph.D.
Caplin and Drysdale
One Thomas Circle, N.W.
Washington, DC 20005

Eugene P. Cronkite, M.D.
Medical Department
Brookhaven National Laboratory
Upton, NY 11973-5000

David A. Crouse, M.D.
University of Nebraska Medical Center
42nd and Dewey Avenue
Omaha, NE 68105

Martin Daly, M.D.
Commander Medical
Headquarters, Northern Ireland
London, England BF PO 801

Neil F. Davies, M.D.
Medical Suite Bedminster Down
Central Electricity Generating Board
Bridgewater Road
Bristol, England B313 8AN

Robert M. DeBell, Ph.D.
Experimental Hematology Department
Armed Forces Radiobiology Research Institute
Bethesda, MD 20814-5145

Robert F. Dons, M.D.
Lt Col, USAF, MC
Box 793
USAF School of Aerospace Medicine
Brooks AFB, TX 78235-5000

Sqn Ldr K. C. Edsall, M.D.
Institute of Naval Medicine
Alverstoke GOSPORT, Hant, England

Thomas B. Elliott, Ph.D.
Experimental Hematology Department
Armed Forces Radiobiology Research Institute
Bethesda, MD 20814-5145

Nushin K. Farzaneh, Ph.D.
Radiation Biochemistry Department
Armed Forces Radiobiology Research Institute
Bethesda, MD 20814-5145

Daniel Flynn, M.D.
74 Wilbur Street
Waltham, MA 02154

Manuel Fuentes, M.D.
Radiotherapy Service
Hospital Militar Gomez ULLA
28047 Madrid, Spain

Reinhard Gahbauer, M.D.
Radiation Oncology
Ohio State University
410 West 10th Avenue
Columbus, OH 45210

Robert P. Gale, M.D.
Division of Hematology/Oncology
Department of Medicine
School of Medicine
University of California
Los Angeles, CA 90024-1678

Richard S. Geary, Ph.D.
Southwest Research Institute
P.O. Drawer 28510
San Antonio, TX 78284

James D. George, Ph.D.
CAPT, MSC, USN
2105 Sheriff Court
Vienna, VA 22180

Joseph P. Geraci, Ph.D.
University of Washington
Radiological Science, SB-75
Seattle, WA 98195

Glenn S. Harmon, M.D.
Department of Medical Oncology
Wilford Hall, USAF Medical Center
Lackland AFB, TX 78236

Erwin Hirsch, M.D.
CAPT, MC, USN
Department of Surgery
Boston University Medical Center
Boston, MA 02118

David Hogg, M.D.
Toronto General Hospital
200 Elizabeth Street
EC 3-306 Toronto, Ontario
M5G 2C4 Canada

Mohammed A. Hussain, M.D.
Veterans Administration Hospital
50 Irving Street, N.E.
Washington, DC 20422

Douglas W. Johnson, M.D.
Baptist Medical Center
8265 Riding Club Road
Jacksonville, FL 32256

Gordon C. Johnson, M.D.
U.S. Food and Drug Administration
1390 Piccard Drive, Suite 300
Rockville, MD 20850

Troyce Jones
Oak Ridge National Laboratory
4500S, F252, M.S. 6106
P.O. Box 2008
Oak Ridge, TN 37831-6101

W. F. J. C. Koster, M.D.
Hoofd Bedrijfsgezondheidsdienst
Westerduinweg 3, Postbus 1
1755 ZG Petten
Netherlands

Dorothee Krumwieh, M.D.
Research Laboratories
Behringwerke AG
P.O. Box 1140
D-3550 Marburg/Lahn
Federal Republic of Germany

K. Sree Kumar, Ph.D.
Radiation Biochemistry Department
Armed Forces Radiobiology Research Institute
Bethesda, MD 20814-5145

Adam Lawson, M.D.
British Nuclear Fuels PLC
Risley, Warrington
Cheshire, England WA3695

Joseph Laver, M.D.
Department of Pediatrics
Medical University of South Carolina
171 Ashley Avenue
Charleston, SC 29425

G. David Ledney, Ph.D
Experimental Hematology Department
Armed Forces Radiobiology Research Institute
Bethesda, MD 20814-5145

Thomas A. Lincoln, M.D.
Oak Ridge Associated Universities
P.O. Box 117
Oak Ridge, TN 37831

Thomas A. Lorance, M.D.
4556 East L. K. Harriet Parkway
Minneapolis, MN 55409-1747

Clarence Lushbaugh, Ph.D., M.D.
Medical and Health Sciences Division
Oak Ridge Associated Universities
Oak Ridge, TN 37831-0117

Thomas J. MacVittie, Ph.D.
Experimental Hematology Department
Armed Forces Radiobiology Research Institute
Bethesda, MD 20814-5145

Kenneth F. McCarthy, Ph.D.
Radiation Biochemistry Department
Armed Forces Radiobiology Research Institute
Bethesda, MD 20814-5145

Patricia Mertz
Department of Dermatology and
    Cutaneous Surgery
School of Medicine
University of Miami
P.O. Box 016250 (R-250)
Miami, FL 33101

G. Andrew Mickley, Ph.D.
Lt Col, USAF, BSC
Radiation Sciences Division
USAF School of Aerospace Medicine (RZP)
Brooks AFB, TX 78235-5301

Robert H. Mosebar, M.D.
Commandant
Academy of Health Sciences (HSHA-DCD)
Fort Sam Houston, TX 78234-6100

Calvin P. Myers, M.D.
3632 NE 72nd Terrace
Gladstone, MO 64119

Alexandre R. Oliveira, M.D.
Institudo Nuclebra de Seguridade Social
Av. Presidente Wilson, 231-8?
Rio de Janeiro, Brazil Cep.:20.030

Graeme R. Peel, M.D.
Wing Commander
Chief, Flight Medicine
HQ TAC/SGPA
Langley AFB, VA 23665

William P. Peters, M.D.
Bone Marrow Transplant Program
Division of Hematology/Oncology
Department of Medicine
Duke University Medical Center
Durham, NC 27701

Madhavan V. Pillai, M.D.
Associate Clinical Professor of Medicine
George Washington University
   Medical Center
Washington, DC 20037

John D. Reardon
Health Resources Services Administration
Public Health Service
Parklawn Bldg., Rm. 14-48
5600 Fishers Lane
Rockville, MD 20857

Robert C. Ricks, Ph.D.
Radiation Emergency Assistance
   Center/Training Site
Medical and Health Sciences Division
P.O. Box 117
Oak Ridge, TN 37831-0117

Roger F. Robison, M.D.
Terre Haute Regional Hospital
20 Cresthill Road
Terre Haute, IN 47802

Henry D. Royal, M.D.
Mallinckrodt Institute of Radiology
510 S. Kingshighway Boulevard
St. Louis, MO 63110

Alfred Rudolph, M.D.
Cetus Corporation
1400 53rd Street
Emeryville, CA 94608

Arnold J. Sattler, M.D.
Holzer Medical Center
203 Jackson Pike
Gallipolis, OH 45631

Stephen C. Schimpff, M.D.
University of Maryland Medical System
Baltimore, MD 21201

James G. Schwade, M.D.
Department of Radiation Oncology
Jackson Memorial North Wing
University of Miami
P.O. Box 016960 (D-31)
Miami, FL 33101

Bobby R. Scott, Ph.D.
Lovelace Inhalation Toxicology
   Research Institute
P.O. Box 5890
Albuquerque, NM 87111

Carol L. Scott, M.D.
Health and Safety Division
Ontario Hydro
700 University Avenue H2D27
Toronto, Ontario M5G 1X6
Canada

Petro Shandruk
U.S. Food and Drug Administration (HFZ-60)
5600 Fishers Lane
Rockville, MD 20857

Torsten Sohns, M.D.
Lt Col, MC, GAF
Federal Ministry of Defense
InSan I 3
D-5300 Bonn, Germany

Rainer Storb, M.D.
Fred Hutchinson Cancer Research Center
1124 Columbia Street
Seattle, WA 98104

C. Robert Valeri, M.D.
Naval Blood Research Laboratory
615 Albany Street
Boston, MA 02118

Howard H. Vogel, Sr., Ph.D.
Biology Department
Memphis State University
280 Ben Avon Way
Memphis, TN 38111

Thomas Walden, Ph.D.
Radiation Biochemistry Department
Armed Forces Radiobiology Research Institute
Bethesda, MD 20814-5145

Richard Walker, Ph.D.
CAPT, MSC, USN
Director, Enteric Diseases
Naval Medical Research Institute
Bethesda, MD 20814-5055

Terry Wall, M.D.
Heart of America Radiation Oncology
5011 Neosho
Shawnee Mission, KS 66205

Thomas Walsh, M.D.
Section of Infectious Diseases
Pediatric Branch
National Cancer Institute
Bethesda, MD 20892

Joseph F. Weiss, Ph.D.
Radiation Biochemistry Department
Armed Forces Radiobiology Research Institute
Bethesda, MD 20814-5145

Catherine D. Williams
MSgt, USAF
Radiation Biochemistry Department
Armed Forces Radiobiology Research Institute
Bethesda, MD 20814-5145

Robert Young, Ph.D.
Radiation Policy Division
Defense Nuclear Agency
Washington, DC 20305-1000

Gary P. Zaloga, M.D.
Department of Anesthesia and Medicine
Bowman Gray School of Medicine
Wake Forest University
Winston-Salem, NC 27103

Small Group Facilitators

Mildred A. Donlon, Ph.D.
Office of the Director
Armed Forces Radiobiology Research Institute
Bethesda, MD 20814-5145

Robert F. Dons, M.D.
Lt Col, USAF, MC
Box 793
USAF School of Aerospace Medicine
Brooks AFB, TX 78235-5000

Pamela J. Gunter-Smith, Ph.D.
Physiology Department
Armed Forces Radiobiology Research Institute
Bethesda, MD 20814-5145

Larry W. Luckett, Ph.D.
LTC, MS, USA
Physics Department
U.S. Military Academy
West Point, NY 10996

G. Andrew Mickley, Ph.D.
Lt Col, USAF, BSC
USAF School of Aerospace Medicine (RZP)
Brooks AFB, TX 78235-5301

Rodney L. Monroy, Ph.D.
LCDR, MSC, USN
Immunobiology and Transplantation Branch
Naval Medical Research Institute
Bethesda, MD 20814-5055

Ruth Neta, Ph.D.
Experimental Hematology Department
Armed Forces Radiobiology Research Institute
Bethesda, MD 20814-5145

Myra L. Patchen, Ph.D.
Experimental Hematology Department
Armed Forces Radiobiology Research Institute
Bethesda, MD 20814-5145

Robert C. Ricks, Ph.D.
Radiation Emergency Assistance
    Center/Training Site
Medical and Health Sciences Division
P.O. Box 117
Oak Ridge, TN 37831-0117

Index

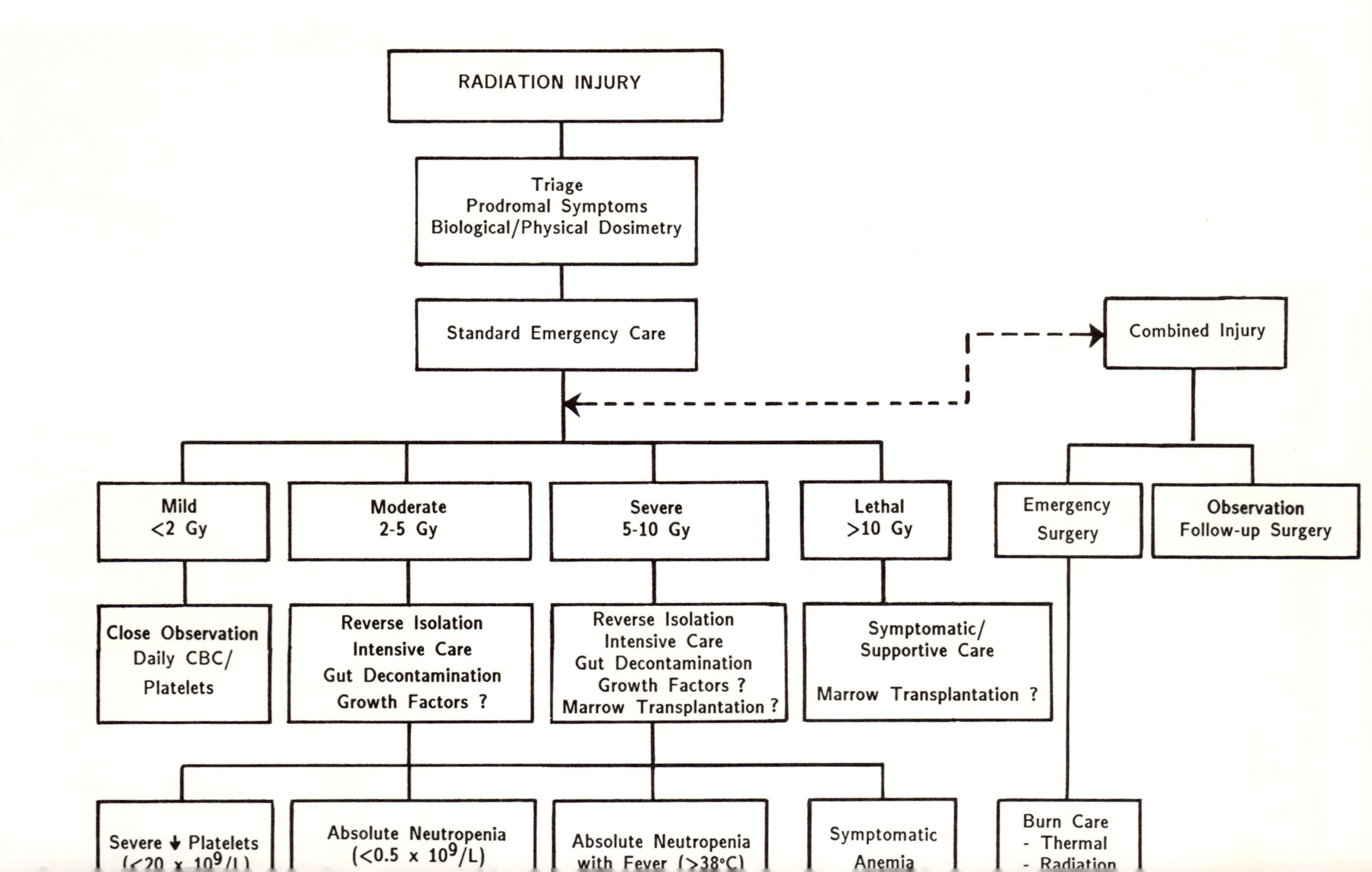

RADIATION INJURY
Triage
Prodromal Symptoms
Biological/Physical Dosimetry
Standard Emergency Care
Combined Injury
Mild
<2 Gy
Moderate
2-5 Gy
Severe
5-10 Gy
Lethal
>10 Gy
Emergency Surgery
Observation
Follow-up Surgery
Close Observation
Daily CBC/
Platelets
Reverse Isolation
Intensive Care
Gut Decontamination
Growth Factors ?
Reverse Isolation
Intensive Care
Gut Decontamination
Growth Factors ?
Marrow Transplantation ?
Symptomatic/
Supportive Care
Marrow Transplantation ?
Severe ↓ Platelets
(<20 x 10⁹/L)
Absolute Neutropenia
(<0.5 x 10⁹/L)
Absolute Neutropenia
with Fever (>38°C)
Symptomatic
Anemia
Burn Care
- Thermal
- Radiation